D1145465

Bv list

The Naked Consultation

A practical guide to primary care consultation skills

Liz Moulton MBE, MBChB, MMEd, FRCGP
GP *and GP trainer, College Lane Surgery, Ackworth*
Associate Director of Postgraduate General Practice Education (Yorkshire)

Foreword by
Roger Neighbour

Radcliffe Publishing
Oxford • Seattle

Radcliffe Publishing Ltd
18 Marcham Road
Abingdon
Oxon OX14 1AA
United Kingdom

www.radcliffe-oxford.com
Electronic catalogue and worldwide online ordering facility.

© 2007 Liz Moulton

Liz Moulton has asserted her right under the Copyright, Designs and Patents Act 1998 to be identified as the author of this work.

All rights reserved. No part of this publication may be reproduced, stored in a retrieval system or transmitted, in any form or by any means, electronic, mechanical, photocopying, recording or otherwise, without the prior permission of the copyright owner.

British Library Cataloguing in Publication Data

A catalogue record for this book is available from the British Library.

ISBN-10: 1 85775 893 5
ISBN-13: 978 185775 893 1

Typeset by Lapiz Digital Services, Chennai
Printed and bound by TJI Digital, Padstow, Cornwall

Contents

Foreword

Liz Moulton comes from what (to me at least!) is a newer generation of hands-on GP trainers and educators. She takes it for granted (in a way that some of her own successors may yet need to be persuaded) that good consulting should be endemic in the general practice community, and has set out to ensure that her own enthusiasm for the consultation is as infectious as possible. Her book is exactly what it says on the tin: *'a practical guide to consultation skills for any health professional working in primary care'*.

We in the UK might modestly claim that ideas from British general practice have, over the last few decades, colonised much of that dark continent of the medical world, 'communication'. During that time, much has been achieved. The maps and models are now pretty well drafted and the territory reasonably comprehensively explored. We are probably past a time when much that is fresh remains to be discovered about what makes an effective consultation. Instead we are now into a period of consolidating, explaining, encouraging – motivating the next generation of GPs to take pride in their own consulting abilities and showing them how to get comfortable with the necessary skills.

In the first part of this book, Liz Moulton presents in her own approachable style the key features of most of the established consultation literature. The second part, of as much interest to teachers and trainers as to clinicians in training, reviews a wide array of current teaching and learning methods. She covers PUNs and DENs, working with colleagues, case discussion, role play and video in eminently practical ways. *The Naked Consultation* is a practical and readable *vademecum* for the would-be skilled consulter.

Roger Neighbour MA, DSc, FRCP, FRCGP
Bedmond
October 2006

About the author

Liz Moulton is a general practitioner (GP) and GP trainer in Ackworth, near Pontefract in West Yorkshire. She is also Associate Director of Postgraduate General Practice Education for Yorkshire.

Liz graduated from Leeds University and was a GP registrar on the Airedale training scheme. She then moved, via Sheffield and New Zealand, to Dundee, where she worked in the Medical School Teaching Practice, before finally settling in Yorkshire. She has been course organiser for the Leeds Vocational Training Scheme for General Practice, has worked in primary care development for Leeds Health Authority and was a GP adviser to the Department of Health. With a life-long interest in the process of consultation, Liz has also run many courses on consultation skills for GPs, GP registrars, nurses and nurse practitioners. She was absolutely delighted to be awarded an MBE in 2005 for services to medicine and healthcare in Yorkshire.

Married to a consultant cardiologist, Liz has three sons, two of whom are medical students.

Acknowledgements

I would like to acknowledge the help and support of many friends and colleagues in, around and beyond the Yorkshire Deanery and, in particular, George Taylor and Brian Ormston, who helped me to get started with *The Naked Consultation* in the first place and were supportive throughout. Thanks also to David Miles, who taught me how to make patients feel better; Jamie Bahrami, who always had faith in me; Mark Purvis, who came up with the title; Alison Evans, who read the final manuscript and made numerous helpful suggestions and corrections; Peter Dickson, John Lord and Richard Sloan, who also read the manuscript and contributed many other suggestions; John Spencer from Newcastle for his unsolicited and most welcome encouragement; Sheena McMain for her creative teaching skills; and Bryce Taylor for everything that I have learnt from him.

My partners at College Lane Surgery, Ackworth – Ivan Hanney, Karen Needham, Jonathan Eastwood and Lisa Yellop – are the best GPs I have ever worked with and the most supportive partners anywhere; I have learnt a lot from each of them, from our GP registrars and, of course, from our patients.

Roger Neighbour's books have had a profound and lasting influence on my own consulting and teaching styles and techniques. I am indebted to him and delighted that he agreed to write the Foreword for this book.

Without the encouragement and behind-the-scenes work of Gillian Nineham and Jamie Etherington at Radcliffe, this book would never have come into being; I am very thankful to them both.

Above all, I would like to thank my family for their tolerance and patience for all that I haven't done over the last two years.

Dedicated to Richard, Andrew, Mike and Robert, with love, and in the hope that, whether as doctors or patients, they may enjoy their future consultations!

Introduction

The Naked Consultation is a practical guide to consultation skills for any health professional working in primary care. This includes GP principals and non-principals, nurses and nurse practitioners and anyone who is currently learning or training in these areas.

Background

When GPs and nurses/nurse practitioners are training, a great deal of time and attention is devoted to their consultation skills – regular debriefing, joint surgeries, video analysis and weekly tutorials. But once these individuals become fully fledged, few have any formal opportunity to reflect further on their consultation skills. It is assumed that they can now consult well enough and will continue to learn 'on the job'.

The consultation, rightly, is a private and intimate interaction between clinician and patient with generally no place for an observer. Even in teaching and training practices, it is relatively unusual for practitioners to sit in on each other's consultations or look together at consultation videos. If you were to ask why, it's likely you would be told that everyone is too busy, there are patients to see and targets to meet. Sitting in or videoing are regarded, at best, as a luxury for which we don't have time and, at worst, completely unnecessary. It is undeniable that most clinicians are busy, but I suspect it isn't the whole truth. The idea of someone watching and commenting on your consultations is quite challenging or even threatening. Even if consultation skills are identified as an important learning area, it can be all too easy for these to get lost, crowded out by all the other demands of modern primary care.

What this means is that most of us have little ongoing experience of 'normative' behaviour. In other words, because there isn't anyone looking over your shoulder, no one challenges you about why you did something in a particular way. Equally, we don't generally watch a colleague's consultation techniques, so can't observe the effect of different tools and styles. So over the years, habits become ingrained, and we consult in a way that 'works for us' and there's nothing wrong with that – most of the time, at least. Sometimes doctors and nurses only really start to think about consultations when something starts to go wrong. This might be a complaint, a clinical error, a systems failure or just increasing tiredness, loss of enjoyment of consultations or the early signs of burnout.

This book is based on a practical handbook written for a Yorkshire Deanery course, developed to meet the needs of those who are no longer officially 'learners' and to enable GP principals and nurses/nurse practitioners to reflect on their consultation skills and enhance them. It also draws on practical experience over many years of teaching GPs, nurses and GP registrars both individually and in groups.

Links to other models

The Naked Consultation relates to a number of different backgrounds, particularly consultation models, such as Neighbour and Calgary–Cambridge, that are focused on process and skills, and also to some counselling frameworks – especially Rogerian (person-centred) counselling, transactional analysis and neurolinguistic programming (NLP).

This book doesn't describe a new model of the consultation process – there are plenty of those already – but it will help you to discover, recognise, practise and extend your own model of the consultation. If there are holes or gaps or fuzzy boundaries, you will be able to identify and deal with them. *The Naked Consultation* emphasises a practical approach – it isn't full of theory or jargon and you don't have to read it from cover to cover in order to make good use of it.

A brief note on language

As the book is for doctors, nurses and others, I have generally used the term 'clinician'. Where I have used the words 'nurse' or 'doctor', these are interchangeable. Similarly, as patients come in both genders, you can usually use 'she' instead of 'he' in your head if you prefer, and vice versa. The word 'consultation' means the interaction between a primary care clinician and their patient and the word 'surgery' means the place where this normally occurs.

Using the book

Like all clinicians, you will have a range of skills you use all the time in many consultations – a toolkit of techniques that work. You probably use some tools frequently, others less often or only rarely. There may be some that have become rusty or discarded and others that were never there in the first place. Using this book will help you identify and polish your existing tools, reuse rusty ones and perhaps add some new ones as well.

The book has two main sections and the chapters within these can be used separately, in any order, as stand-alone modules, or as part of an integrated whole. Some clinicians may want to dip into the parts of the book that meet their immediate problems or needs (for example, after a difficult consultation) and may go straight to the relevant chapter. Others may take a more structured approach and use the book to reflect on their consultation style and skills. There are prompts and suggestions throughout, asking you to think about real consultations and consider what you might do in the future. This is to try and make the book as practical and useful as possible and so that you can personalise it and make links and connections with your own consultations.

The two sections are:

Part 1: Deconstructing the consultation

The first part of the book takes the consultation apart and looks in detail at the various phases of the process of consultation. It explores the tools and skills that will help make consultations more effective and efficient.

Part 2: Tools and techniques for learning and improving consultation skills

The second part describes educational tools – such as videoing, random case analysis, problem case debriefing and feedback – to improve consultations. It also explores the MRCGP exam, the requirements of summative assessment and appraisal.

Appendix 1 is a 'jargon buster' for quick and easy reference, and Appendix 2 contains useful, photocopiable forms.

Part 1

Deconstructing the consultation

Prologue

Where am I going, where have I been? Where have I been, where am I going?

(Circular inscription on a handmade plate given to RCGP Yorkshire District Faculty Tutors at a memorable seminar at Hazlewood Castle, Tadcaster in 1992)

Learning consultation skills

I'd like you to think back to the time when you first learnt to consult in primary care. What do you remember? Just cast your mind back for a few moments. Perhaps you remember:

- watching others consult, by sitting in on their surgeries
- trying out consultations for yourself and talking about them with a trainer, mentor or senior colleague
- having a colleague or teacher sit in with you to watch your surgeries and give you feedback.

If it was within the last 15 years or so, you may also remember:

- videoing surgeries
- joint surgeries where you and a mentor or trainer undertook alternate consultations
- debriefing videoed surgeries with a senior colleague
- surgeries with simulated patients.

You may also have received some formal or informal teaching about consultation skills – perhaps on a course with others at the same stage of learning (for example, a half-day release scheme). You might have undertaken some sort of formal assessment process of your consultation skills – by producing a video of a series of consultations or taking part in a simulated patient surgery.

We don't often think about consultations as being a learning experience when we are in the role of patient or relative of a patient, but many health professionals have learnt about aspects of the consultation (both positive and negative) when they have been on the receiving end. These first-hand experiences can be very powerful learning tools.

Example

Jane, a 20-year-old medical student, went to see her GP with a slightly embarrassing problem. She walked into the room, and sat down in the patient's chair, which was directly across the desk. Jane waited anxiously whilst the doctor completed writing the notes of the previous patient and then took out Jane's notes. He skimmed them and then, without looking up at her, opened the consultation with a statement: 'You've come for the Pill.' (She hadn't.) A powerful example, recalled and related many years later, of how not to start a consultation!

However you learnt in the first place, the way you consult now will be different from how it was then. It will have evolved and developed in a way that is unique to you.

Thinking back to when you first learnt to consult, you may remember finding the process difficult or challenging, with lots of different things to think about all at the same time. As you read this book and think about and try some of the suggestions, some of these feelings may re-emerge and your consultations may feel less fluent for a while. This is normal and temporary! It's a bit like driving a car for years and then going on a course to be an advanced driver; you have to go back to the stage of what's called 'conscious competence' before you can start to assimilate new skills into your repertoire. After a few weeks of this, your skills will start to improve again, not just to the level that you started at, but to a much higher level.

Let's stick with the driving analogy for a moment. When you learnt to drive, you may well have experienced the following stages.

Unconscious incompetence

Whenever you see someone carrying out a skilled task, apparently with little effort, it can appear very straightforward and it is easy to underestimate the skills involved.

> Driving is dead easy. Even my mum can do it, so it can't be difficult. You just get in the car and off you go. I'll be 17 soon – I can't wait to get out there. I'll pass my test within a month.

Conscious incompetence

Of course, once you try, it becomes very obvious that it is much more difficult than you thought and the initial overconfidence can be knocked.

> Help – this is quite hard really. So many things to think about at the same time – steering in a straight line, speed, changing gear, looking in your mirror, watching for pedestrians. How come all these idiots can drive and I can't?

Conscious competence

If you keep going and persist through this difficult stage, there comes a time when you, too, can do it, but you have to make a real effort and think carefully about each step of the process.

> Check and adjust the seat position. Make sure the handbrake is on and the gear in neutral. Look in the rear view mirror for traffic and wait until it's clear. Clutch down, first gear, a few revs. Indicate right. Check the blind spot. Bring the clutch up slowly, handbrake off, move forward ...

Unconscious competence

When you practise the skills until they are fluent, you can perform them with much less conscious thought.

I don't really have to think about the clutch and changing gear and indicating and all that any more. It just comes automatically, so I can concentrate much better on the traffic and the road conditions.

Learning new skills

Right now, you may be anywhere along the spectrum from unconscious incompetence to unconscious competence. For example, if you have only recently started learning to consult, you may well be conscious of your competence at times and conscious of your incompetence at others. If you have been consulting for years, your consultation skills will be unconsciously competent. In other words you don't have to think too hard about what you are doing most of the time. If this applies to you, then in order to add new skills, you will need to temporarily go back to the stage of conscious competence.

Whatever stage you are at, new skills that you learn and practise may feel awkward for a while, but will soon get incorporated into your 'unconsciously competent' toolkit.

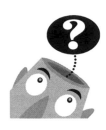

Chapter 1

Consultations – the good, the bad and the difficult

Key points

- It's relatively easy to label a consultation as being 'good', 'bad' or 'difficult', but it can be harder to work out what it is that makes them so.
- We tend to think about difficult consultations as being a problem for us, the clinicians – but they are often equally uncomfortable for our patients.
- Conscious awareness of potholes and pitfalls can help practitioners to do something about them before the consultation goes really badly wrong.

The good

What makes a good consultation? If you ask a number of clinicians you will get as many different answers. Here are some common themes that most clinicians recognise as making a good (not necessarily the same as 'easy') consultation.

- The patient presents a single straightforward problem that you are able to recognise and treat appropriately.
- The patient presents difficult or puzzling symptoms and you are able to make sense of these.
- You are able to give some added value to the consultation, such as remembering to advise the patient to stop smoking, and they seem to listen and take on board what you say.
- A result comes back confirming a suspected diagnosis – and it's something that's straightforward to treat, will make a real difference to how the patient feels and it's not life threatening (for example, hypothyroidism).
- Every patient in a morning's surgery has something that you can help with and you keep to time.

What about patients? When you read patient satisfaction surveys, it is clear what patients value in consultations.

> 'The doctor/nurse/healthcare practitioner really listened to me.'
> 'I felt that the doctor understood me.'
> 'I had enough time with the doctor/nurse.'
> 'The doctor/nurse really explained things in a way that I could understand.'

The bad

From a clinician's perspective, bad consultations can include the following.

- The consultation starts badly and never really recovers.

- You don't have the really significant new piece of information that the patient assumes you do have (for example, a new diagnosis of cancer).
- You discover late in the consultation that you have a completely different patient in front of you from the one you expected – the 'wrong' patient has come into the room.
- You only obtain a crucial piece of information very late on and after you have formulated a management plan (which is now completely wrong).
- Strong emotions such as anger (yours, the patient's or both) start to predominate and get in the way of effective consulting.

What do patients say?

> 'I felt rushed – the doctor didn't seem to have time for me.'
> 'The doctor didn't listen.'
> 'The doctor used words I didn't understand.'
> 'I felt patronised.'
> 'He didn't seem to know what he was doing.'

... and the difficult

So what causes difficulties in consultations? Quite clearly, there are some consultations that are always going to be difficult because of the nature of the problem. Examples are:

- you have to break bad news to a patient
- the patient comes in very angry
- the patient comes with a list of several problems, some or all of which are potentially significant.

These are consultations which get (a bit) easier with practice and where you can improve your skills by practice, reflection and rehearsal, but which are always going to be challenging.

There are many 'ordinary' consultations, though, that feel more difficult than you would expect. On some days, you feel exhausted at the end of surgery and yet, when you think back, there were no particularly stressful or difficult consultations – it just seems to be an accumulation of a lot of different, relatively minor factors that have got on top of you and perhaps eroded your capacity to consult effectively. You may have found yourself longing for a late cancellation, a 'Did Not Attend' (DNA), a real 'quickie' or just the end of the surgery.

It can be a chain reaction; one difficult consultation leads to another ... and another .... For example, if you haven't been able to get rid of all the negative feelings that you have been left with at the end of a complex or emotionally laden consultation, these feelings may persist and start interfering with, and hampering, your subsequent consultations. A common consequence of having several consultations with minor difficulties in a row is that you can start to run late. This can make things even worse if you try to catch up.

- The patient who has been kept waiting for 20 minutes or even longer is now determined to have their full 10 minutes' worth and to make sure you don't rush them.

- Whilst waiting to see you, the patient has been thinking about their health and has recalled several additional problems that they would like you to deal with today.
- You may try and cut corners and miss significant areas of the consultation – moving into the management plan before the patient has had a chance to tell you what they had in mind themselves can add significant minutes of back-tracking, delay and frustration for clinician and patient.
- Your capacity for consulting effectively may have been eroded and you may ignore or miss patient cues leading to a dysfunctional consultation.

Activity

Think about consultations you have had over the last week or two. Try to identify:
A 'good' consultation

- What made it good?
- What skills did you use?
- How did you feel at the end of it?

A 'bad' consultation

- What made it bad – bad for you or the patient, or both?
- What might you have done differently?
- How did you feel at the end of it?

A 'difficult' consultation

- What made it difficult?
- How was it different from the bad consultation?
- How did you feel at the end of it?

Potholes and pitfalls

So what makes some consultations more difficult than others? There are four key areas and any combination of two or three of these can turn a mildly difficult consultation into a really awful one – usually for both the clinician and the patient. These are the key areas.

- You, the clinician
- Patient factors
- The relationship between you and the patient
- Extraneous factors.

You, the clinician

Sometimes you know perfectly well that you're not in good shape even before the surgery starts. Perhaps you:

- were working for the out-of-hours service, out at a party or just slept badly
- had to drive through really bad traffic to get to the surgery

- had a row with your spouse before you set out
- have other problems at home that are troublesome and intrusive
- are feeling ill or below par
- have just had some personal bad news
- haven't had a holiday for a while
- or are just back from holiday and not really in consultation mode yet.

At other times, the surgery started out fine, but has subsequently become chaotic or out of hand, perhaps due to:

- running late
- a series of complex consultations
- a really difficult consultation that has left you angry, hurt or upset – and you haven't been able to manage or even 'park' these feelings so they are still hanging around you.

Patient factors

It's the same with patients; they, too, frequently come into the consulting room with emotional baggage. Like you, they may be tired, have had a row, need a holiday or have driven through bad traffic. They may also:

- be angry or upset for some reason that's nothing to do with you
- have been kept waiting a long time without explanation so that any emotions such as anxiety or anger will have increased in intensity during the wait
- have completely unreasonable expectations of the clinician and the consultation
- have a list of several problems
- be very anxious about what's wrong but displace this feeling into anger, irritability or unreasonable behaviour.

At other times, as with the doctor, the consultation has started out fine but has then degenerated because the patient perhaps:

- does not feel listened to
- perceives that their fears are ignored or inadequately addressed
- feels they are being rushed
- takes a dislike to you.

The relationship between clinician and patient

Sometimes the difficulty seems to lie in the relationship between the clinician and the patient. This is often due to communication difficulties of various sorts including the following situations.

- The clinician and patient misunderstand each other because they are trying to communicate without a shared language in which both are fluent.
- The clinician or patient has difficulty understanding the strong regional accent or dialect, or misinterprets the meaning of words used by the other. This can include colloquial words used by the patient and, of course, the 'medical speak' that we may use inadvertently when talking with patients.

> I did all my GP training in Yorkshire. When my husband's career led to a move to Dundee, I found that I had to concentrate on every word that the patients said just to understand the meaning; patients' accents and use of words that I had never heard before made consulting much more difficult at first:
>
> 'eh' – 'I'
> 'peely wally' – 'washed out'
> 'twa' – 'two'
> 'wabbit' – 'not at all well'

- The patient (or clinician) has poor hearing.

The difficulty can also be due to differing ideas and expectations about what will happen in the consultation. For example:

- The patient who is genuinely expecting a prescription will be taken aback by the clinician who 'only' offers advice and whom they therefore perceive to have 'done nothing'.
- The clinician or patient (or both) may carry memories of a previous consultation together and unhelpfully project these into the current one. This can also happen when a patient has had a difficult consultation with a completely different clinician, but brings their frustrations or negative feelings into the here-and-now of today's consultation with you.

Extraneous factors

Sometimes, aspects of the consulting room can have a negative influence.

- The room is too cold, hot, dark, noisy or unwelcoming.
- Distractions in the room intrude into the consultation:
  - visual distractions, such as eye-catching photographs or unusual art
  - auditory distractions, such as sounds from the waiting room, the consulting room next door or traffic going past
  - olfactory distractions, such as the lingering smell of garlic or the body odour of previous patients.
- Seating arrangements are sub-optimal:
  - the patient's chair is hard or uncomfortable
  - the patient's chair is lower than the doctor's
  - seats that are on opposite sides of the desk (a bit like the bank manager's).
- There are interruptions from:
  - the telephone
  - the doctor's (or patient's) mobile phone ringing
  - people coming in (for example, nurses to get prescriptions signed, receptionists with coffee, the registrar with a problem patient who can't wait, the patient who was actually looking for the consulting room next door).

- The computer intrudes:
  - the clinician struggles with the 'needs' of the computer
  - the patient perceives that the clinician pays more attention to the needs of the computer than their own needs
  - the computer crashes or freezes during the consultation and needs to be reset
  - sub-optimal positioning of the computer (for example, so that it can only be read by the doctor and not the patient, or is placed so that the doctor needs to turn away to look at it)
  - the printer is out of paper or the paper jams whilst the prescription is being printed. Then it does it again!

Have you ever looked at your consulting room from the patient's point of view? If you haven't, it can be enlightening to knock on the door, walk in and sit down in your own patient's chair.

- What do you see as you walk across the room?
- How comfortable is the patient's chair when you sit down?
- What is the relative height of the two chairs? If the patient's chair is lower than the clinician's, then the patient may consciously or unconsciously feel at a disadvantage right from the start – this does nothing to empower them or help them manage their own health and symptoms.
- What view do you have from this chair?
- Can you read the computer screen or is it hidden from view? If it is turned away from you (the patient) – how does it feel? Wouldn't you be curious to see what the clinician was typing about you?

You could ask someone else's opinion about this too – a colleague in the practice or a receptionist. One way of doing this would be to take a photograph of the view from the patient's chair. Show it to a colleague and ask what they see.

Overall, how do you think it feels to be the patient in your consultation? What could you do to improve this from the patient's point of view?

Possible action points

- Over the next week or two, notice which consultations seem to be particularly draining or stressful, and make a note of them. Can you identify any themes or patterns? Do these consultations tend to contain doctor, patient, extraneous or relationship difficulties?
- Have a good, objective look at your consulting room (perhaps with a colleague – ideally one who isn't familiar with the room from the patient's perspective). Is it arranged optimally for both you and the patient? Are there any steps that you could take to improve it?
- When you do become stressed in a consultation, think about what (if anything) you already do to improve how you're feeling. Make a few notes about this.

Further reading

- Tate P. *The Doctor's Communication Handbook*. 5th edn. Oxford: Radcliffe Publishing; 2007.

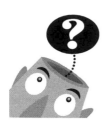

Chapter 2

Models and milestones

Medicine is an enormous model shop in which to browse, occupying as it does the common ground between mankind's physical, mental and spiritual experiences.

Neighbour (1987)

Key points

- A model is just a way of describing any task that you do, or have done, more than once.
- There are numerous books describing different consultation models, most of them aimed at doctors, but just as suitable for nurses and other health professionals.
- Some models are more focused on what needs to be achieved during the consultation (the task) and others are more about how this happens (the process).
- Some models are more focused on the clinician and others on the patient's perspective.
- All models are partial or incomplete – they can't possibly describe every aspect of every consultation.

Many books describing different consultation models have been written. The models have similarities and differences, and areas that overlap. Thinking about consultation models can be a useful way of putting a framework or structure on your own model of the consultation (i.e. the way that you yourself consult most fluently and competently). Sometimes looking at a particular model and seeing how it is different from your own can prompt you to adjust and modify your own consultation process.

Why bother with 'models' at all?

A model is just a description of how we do something. Each of us has our own model (whether or not we choose to think of it as such, or give it a name) for almost everything that we have done more than once. You will have a model, for example, for:

- waking up and getting out of bed
- making and eating a meal
- getting the car out and driving to work
- going into the surgery and greeting the staff

... and for just about everything else that you do during an ordinary day.

Even a very straightforward action such as pouring a glass of water will have a model, and yours will be slightly different from mine or from anyone else's. In its simplest and most stripped-down form, my model might sound as if it is very like yours.

open cupboard → take out glass → turn on tap → pour in water until glass is nearly full → turn off tap

But the details will be different. Which cupboard? Where is it? How does it open? Which glass do you choose? How do you take the glass out? Which hand do you use? How long do you run the tap? Do you use a water cooler or bottled water?

Exploring the edges of the model is useful because it can help to uncover unconscious presumptions. For example, I might assume that you would turn on the cold tap and nearly fill the glass with cold water because this is what I do and what I have done hundreds of times before – but it is just an assumption. If I discovered that you actually poured a glass of hot water or that you only half-filled the glass, or that you only ever drank Perrier, I might be surprised, and compare what you do with what I do. I could then choose to try out what you do, or even permanently change what I do, or I might decide that my way is better after all!

Thinking about the consultation, I might particularly want to change if my current behaviour causes me problems, makes me feel stressed or just doesn't seem to work very well. In other words, reading about or exploring a previously described model of the consultation would help me to identify my own model and reflect on it. This might be something that I would not otherwise have done.

Consultation models

As with pouring a glass of water, every health professional has their own model of the consultation – you have yours and I have mine, and most of the time they work, more or less. Ever since your first consultation, you will have been building and refining your own consultation model. It's likely this model works well enough most of the time, but what about when you have a difficult or unusual consultation? Do you want to explore the 'edges' of your model and think about whether to refine, change or modify them?

Looking at and playing with models described by others can help make sense of your own model – is it similar to one of the others or very different? Are there good bits of other models that you could borrow and add to yours?

Similarities between models

All consultation models have two key similarities.

- They are partial or incomplete – in other words they don't and can't describe everything to do with every permutation of consultation.
- Most of them include each of the following five key stages:
  - find out why the patient has come
  - work out what's wrong
  - explain the problem(s) to the patient
  - develop a management plan for the patient's problem(s)
  - use the time well and efficiently.

Some models explicitly include a sixth and very important stage – look after yourself so that you stay in good shape.

Some models are more focused on the tasks of the consultation – in other words, what needs to be achieved by the clinician. Others are more concerned with the process of consultation. Both task and process are important and, like the yin and yang, together they make a complete whole (*see* Figure 2.1).

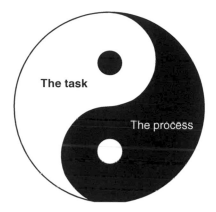

Figure 2.1 Yin and yang

The tasks of the consultation

Some models are more about the clinician and others are more patient-centred. For example:

The traditional medical interview

This is an example of a doctor-centred, task-focused consultation process:

- patient presents symptoms
- doctor asks questions and examines patient
- doctor pronounces diagnosis and/or treatment
- patient goes away.

The Pendleton model of the consultation

This is another task-focused model, but more patient-centred than the traditional medical interview. The seven tasks to be achieved are:

- **First task** Find out why the patient has come, including the problem (cause, effects, history) and the patient's ideas, concerns and expectations.
- **Second task** Consider other problems.
- **Third task** Choose (with the patient) an appropriate action for each problem.
- **Fourth task** Achieve a shared understanding of the problems.
- **Fifth task** Involve the patient in the management and encourage them to accept appropriate responsibility.
- **Sixth task** Use time and resources appropriately.
- **Seventh task** Establish or maintain a relationship with the patient which helps to achieve the other tasks.

This model moves away from the doctor-centeredness of earlier models and does at least include the patient in tasks 3, 4 and 5. But it is very task-focused, and it isn't until the seventh task that the relationship with the patient gets a mention!

The Helman folk model

This is a much more patient-centred model. Cecil Helman, a medical anthropologist, suggests that any patient comes to a doctor seeking answers to six questions:

1. What has happened?
2. Why has it happened?
3. Why to me?
4. Why now?
5. What would happen if nothing was done about it?
6. What should I do about it or whom should I consult for further help?

In other words, all patients have questions that they would like you to answer. Sometimes the questions are clearly expressed, but at other times they are not – they may be hidden or not asked. To be effective, the clinician may need to help the patient verbalise these questions so they can be addressed.

Milestones in the development of the process of consultation

There have been some key steps on the pathway to the primary care consultation process.

The Doctor, his Patient and the Illness

Michael Balint and his wife, Enid, were Hungarian psychoanalysts who emigrated to the UK in the 1930s and did ground-breaking work with GPs in London in the 1950s and 1960s, reported in the classic book, *The Doctor, his Patient and the Illness* (1957). (This was at a time when most doctors were men and most consultations lasted, at most, six minutes.) They helped groups of GPs to explore the psychological aspects of their consultations, at first by encouraging long consultations with patients, but later by fitting small interventions into 'ordinary' consultations.

In their book, they describe significant insights into the primary care consultation.

- Clinician and patient develop an emotional relationship during the consultation.
- Sometimes clinicians and patients collude about what to tackle in the consultation (for example, the clinician who has a problem with alcohol use may choose to ignore cues or hints from the patient about the patient's problem with alcohol).
- As in psychoanalysis, the feelings that arise in a clinician during a consultation may well be coming from the patient. So the clinician who can tune in to their own feelings can use these to help work out what the patient is feeling in the consultation (counter transference).
- Attentive listening helps patients feel better (even if not much else changes). By listening to the clinicians in their groups, they modelled good behaviour and taught the clinicians that good listening helps patients (or their doctors!) to feel better.
- The clinician is one of the most powerful therapeutic agents in the consultation (the doctor as drug).
- A sick or troubled parent (usually the mother) may present their (well) child or baby as the 'symptom' (the child as the presenting complaint).

- Some consultations extend over a period of years and both patient and doctor invest their time and attention in this process, building up a bank of resources, trust and understanding (mutual investment company).
- The clinician may have a 'magician-like' function and be perceived (either by themselves, the patient or both) as holding all the answers up their sleeves (the apostolic function of the doctor).
- Doctors who ask a lot of questions in the consultation get answers to their questions and no more. Balint commented that until a doctor learnt to listen, he would not be able to find out any further useful information. He described listening as a new skill that the doctor would need to learn, requiring a change in the doctor's personality (asking questions only gets you answers).

Byrne and Long

Moving on, Byrne and Long (1976) undertook a large and very significant study of what goes on in consultations. They had a hunch that there was more to consultations than mere illness. This was at a time when, as they report, most medical men showed strong resistance to anything psychological or behavioural which, for most of them, was something to do with rats and pigeons.

They tape-recorded and then analysed 2,500 consultations generated by almost 100 doctors in the UK and New Zealand and discovered that many doctors appeared to lack the tools to deal effectively with the psychological or social aspects of the consultation.

Reporting their findings in *Doctors Talking to Patients* (note 'to' rather than 'with' and 'talking' rather than 'listening'), they described a six-part model. This was evidence-based in that it was developed from observations of a large number of consultations. It is, therefore, solid and well-grounded, but does feel a bit old-fashioned and dated now. It is a product of its time; in the 1970s most consultations lasted no more than six minutes, the number of patients seen in a surgery was almost certainly more than is common now and the visiting rate was much higher. It is understandable that most doctors were trying to hurry their patients. This may well explain why a lot of the consultations described are quite doctor-centred and that their model focuses on what the doctor does. The patient doesn't seem to have a particularly active role in the consultation process at all.

Byrne and Long described six stages in their model.

1. The doctor establishes a relationship with the patient.
2. The doctor attempts to discover or actually discovers the reason for the patient's attendance.
3. The doctor conducts a verbal or physical examination, or both.
4. The doctor alone, the doctor and patient together, or the patient alone (in that order of probability) consider(s) the condition.
5. The doctor, and occasionally the patient, details the treatment or further investigation.
6. The consultation is ended, usually by the doctor.

Analysing these consultations, Byrne and Long made some interesting observations.

- Individual doctors did not have much of a repertoire of consultation skills, but tended to use the same well-worn techniques with all patients. In other words, the doctors tended to stick with a 'model' that they were comfortable with and that they perceived suited both them and their patients. They kept on using the usual tools from their consultation toolkit and could, perhaps, do with some new ones!

- Byrne and Long describe the section of the consultation that comes just after the patient's initial response to the doctor's opening as being one of the most significant parts of the consultation. A shorter stage 2 than average was a key marker for the consultation going adrift. This is not all that surprising; if the doctor does not actually discover the patient's agenda or even why they're there, then the consultation is quite likely to become dysfunctional.
- Patients felt better in consultations that were more patient-centred. Although this might seem obvious now, it was new information at the time.
- Doctors who asked more open questions tended to see their patients less frequently.
- Doctors often misinterpreted non-verbal communication.

Neighbour

Roger Neighbour (1987), in one of the most widely known and significant books on the consultation ever written, *The Inner Consultation*, describes an intuitive five-stage model, which any doctor can adapt to improve the quality of their consultations. It is 'anchored' to the fingers and thumb of the left hand (*see* Figure 2.2).

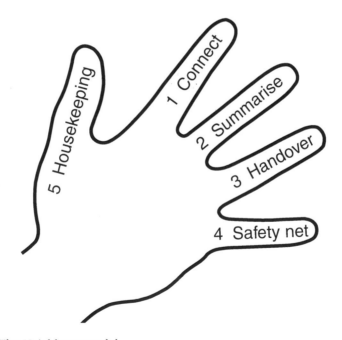

Figure 2.2 The Neighbour model

It is a highly process-orientated model and describes many skills at each of five key stages of the consultation, which Neighbour likens to a journey with way points. The five stages are:

1. **Connecting** Neighbour emphasises the importance of developing rapport with the patient, starting with the first few moments of the consultation and

continuing right through it. This helps the clinician to tune in to the patient, get on the same wavelength and achieve empathy. Once rapport is established, the clinician explores the patient's story and gathers enough information about what is going on to enable them to make a summary.

2. **Summarising** This is a stage of the consultation that had not formed part of previously described models, but is now recognised by many clinicians as being extremely useful. At this point, the patient's reasons for attending, hopes, feelings, concerns and expectations have been explored and acknowledged well enough. The clinician checks this out with the patient.

3. **Handing over** This describes the joint production of an agreed management plan and transfer of control back to the patient.

4. **Safety-netting** A three-part safety net gives both clinician and patient some security; it means there are contingency plans in case the clinician is wrong and/or something unexpected happens.

5. **Housekeeping** This stage recognises the importance of the clinician staying in good shape. It gives the clinician the opportunity to deal with any negative feelings or stress that have arisen during the consultation before the next patient arrives in the room.

The Neighbour model has two key differences from much of the earlier work in consultations.

- **Summarising** is an extremely useful stage that really helps to make sure that the patient has said everything that they need to say, that the doctor is clear about this, and has communicated this effectively to the patient. It also acts as the fulcrum or pivotal point of the consultation, which helps it to move from information gathering to shared planning. If you are ever really stuck in a consultation – summarise!

- **Housekeeping** is now a very familiar part of consultation skills language. Most doctors now recognise how important it is to look after themselves during and after consultations, as well as long-term. Until Neighbour's book, doctors and nurses tended to pay token attention to this. Here, it becomes a key stage of the consultation – as important as finding out why the patient has come.

The Calgary–Cambridge approach

Jonathan Silverman, Suzanne Kurtz and Juliet Draper (1998) have developed an evidence-based and evolving consultation framework that is also very practical. It describes the skills needed at each stage of the consultation in order to improve communication between clinician and patient. It is another five-stage model.

1. **Initiating the session**
   - establishing initial rapport
   - identifying reasons for the consultation
   - negotiating an agenda that includes both the patient's and the clinician's needs.

2. **Gathering information**
   - encouraging the patient to tell their story and to explain 'why now?'
   - using open and closed questions to explore the problem
   - noticing both verbal and non-verbal cues

- finding out ideas, concerns and expectations
- providing structure to the consultation.

3. **Building the relationship**

- development of rapport
- recording notes unobtrusively
- accepting the legitimacy of the patient's view and feelings
- demonstrating sensitivity, empathy and support, thinking aloud.

4. **Explanation and planning**

- giving information in digestible chunks
- checking understanding
- timing explanations carefully so that, for example, reassurance is not given too early
- using diagrams, models and written information to help explanation.

5. **Closing the session**

- summarising
- clarifying the agreed plan.

The Calgary–Cambridge books are comprehensive and packed full of useful skills for primary care consultations.

Narrative-based primary care

John Launer (2002), a London GP and Senior Lecturer in General Practice at the Tavistock Clinic, describes the use of a 'narrative-based' model of consulting. 'Narrative' is a word that we normally use about telling stories and is a very interesting word to use in the context of the consultation. Every primary care clinician is familiar with the fact that most patients don't come in and present a logical and coherent set of symptoms. Instead we see patients with unsifted and unsorted problems and so there tends to be an eclectic mixture that includes:

- some symptoms that may go together and form a pattern
- some that don't fit easily
- the family and social situation
- the patient's past experience of their own illnesses or those of family members
- etc, etc.

So narrative-based medicine acknowledges that people create or write stories in their heads in order to make sense of what has happened, and then tell these stories to other people. Like all stories, they get slightly modified in the process of 'telling'. Patients usually describe their experience in a way that slightly distorts what actually happened. They don't do this deliberately; it's an unconscious way of processing and making sense. All of us do this – if you ever hear someone describing what happened at an event where you were also present (for example, a football match, party or concert) you may well hear quite a different version of the event from the one you experienced. The bare bones may be the same, but the detail of the content will be different.

In consultations, the 'absolute' truth rarely matters and what is much more interesting and useful is what the patient believes to be the truth – which is just as well, as it is usually the only information that we have!

Launer describes some extremely useful techniques for helping to understand patients' stories. For example:

- **Circular questioning** The idea here is to get away from the linear concept of cause and effect, and instead help the patient to focus on meaning, or the problem within the context of the family, for example, picking up the words that the patient has used and then using them to form open questions.
- **Focusing on listening** For example, not making any notes until the end of the consultation.
- **Context** When patients come to see primary healthcare practitioners, there is clearly a medical context to the problem. But there may also be other contexts such as the family, the workplace, faith community or other clinicians that the patient has seen. When a problem doesn't make medical sense, it is well worth finding out about the other contexts.
- **Creating a joint story** Of course, the patient is not the only person in the consultation who tells stories. Doctors, too, have contexts and stories of their own and, as part of the process of consultation both doctor and patient can develop a new and joint story. This helps to emphasise the equality of the relationship between clinician and patient.
- **The power balance** Launer describes deliberately shifting the balance of power in the consultation so that the patient has more of it than is typical.
- **Geneograms** Constructing a family tree with the patient can help doctors to understand the contexts of a patient's problems much better. For example, it may reveal stories from the past that are still weaving their spell in the patient's present.

Consulting with NLP (neurolinguistic programming)

In 2002, Lewis Walker, a GP in Buckie, Scotland, published *Consulting with NLP,* the first of two very readable, well-written and comprehensive guides to using NLP in the consultation. NLP offers a rich vein of tools and techniques to help clinicians to achieve excellent communication with their patients. Many of the techniques in *The Naked Consultation* have their foundation in NLP.

As well as providing an excellent and full guide to NLP for those who are new to the techniques, Walker also links this very clearly to his work and experience as a GP and so provides really useful and very practical tools and techniques for making a difference to communicating with patients.

For anyone with even the slightest interest in the use of NLP in the consultation, this is a must-read book.

Possible action points

- Think about how you consult at the moment. What stages are in your model? Can you describe your own model of the consultation so that another person could follow and replicate it? Are there any potentially useful steps that you tend to leave out at the moment?
- Is your style more doctor-centred or more patient-centred?
- Who does most of the talking? You or the patient?
- Do you tend to be more concerned with achieving the tasks of the consultation or the process of getting there?
- What would you like to change about your model of the consultation?

References and further reading

- Balint M. *The Doctor, his Patient and the Illness.* London: Pitman Medical; 1957. 2nd edn Edinburgh: Churchill Livingstone; 1964, reprinted 1986.
- Byrne PS, Long BEL. *Doctors Talking to Patients.* London: HMSO; 1976.
- Helman CG. Disease versus illness in general practice. *J Royal College of General Practitioners.* 1981; **31:** 548–52.
- Launer J. *Narrative Based Primary Care: a practical guide.* Oxford: Radcliffe Medical Press; 2002.
- Neighbour R. *The Inner Consultation.* Lancaster: MTP Press; 1987. 2nd edn Oxford: Radcliffe Publishing; 2004.
- Pendleton D, Schofield T, Tate P, Havelock P. *The Consultation: an approach to learning and teaching.* Oxford: Oxford University Press; 1984.
- Silverman J, Kurtz S, Draper J. *Skills for Communicating with Patients.* Oxford: Radcliffe Medical Press; 1998. 2nd edn; 2004.
- Walker L. *Consulting with NLP.* Oxford: Radcliffe Medical Press; 2002.
- www.skillscascade.com
- www.gp-training.net

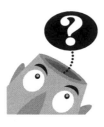

Chapter 3

In the beginning

What we call the beginning is often the end
And to make an end is to make a beginning.
The end is where we start from ...
... We shall not cease from exploration
And the end of all our exploring
Will be to arrive where we started
And know the place for the first time.

'Little Gidding', TS Eliot*

Key points

- Good beginnings make for good consultations!
- There are many different ways of starting a consultation and one of the most effective is to let the patient start it.
- The early minutes of a consultation may well provide most of the information needed to understand the patient and help them effectively.

How do your consultations begin? Have you ever thought about it? Does it matter? They just begin, don't they?

Introduction

Byrne and Long (1976) likened the start of a consultation to two soldiers in the battlefield on Christmas Day. The armies have been there for weeks or months. It's cold, wet and miserable. Rations are low and Christmas dinner is not up to much. The soldiers are all badly missing their homes and families. Each side is well dug into their trenches and, quite frankly, neither side wishes to have a battle or shooting match that day. They would really like to get up out of the trenches and at least stretch their legs in the muddy battle ground. On the other hand, neither side wants to be shot at and killed, and each is quite unclear about the intentions of the other. It's something of a dilemma.

So what do they do? How do they find out the other side's intentions? Well, one of the soldiers raises a small balloon, rather tentatively, just above the level of the parapet and watches to see what happens. Is it going to be shot down? If it is, then at least the intentions of the other party are clear. But if the other side reciprocates and raises another small balloon, then it is clear that, at least for today, it may be possible to play a different game.

The learning here is that the early moments of the consultation are crucial. Patients can be very unsure about what they will tell you and, if they don't know you well, may be completely unable to anticipate how you will

---

*Reproduced with permission of Faber and Faber Ltd from *Collected Poems 1909–1962* by TS Eliot.

respond to a difficult or sensitive matter. If the patient raises a small balloon, figuratively speaking, then make sure you don't inadvertently shoot it down.

The golden minutes

Clinicians in secondary care talk about the 'golden hour' – when dealing with a patient who has suffered severe trauma, for example in an accident. Getting the patient to the trauma room or operating theatre within this window of time optimises the chances of the patient's survival.

In primary care, it can be useful to think about the 'golden minutes' – the two or three minutes at the start of a consultation. Used well, these can give you almost all the information that you need to manage a patient's problems and build the therapeutic relationship. Used badly, the time can simply be wasted or actively impair the developing relationship.

Beginning your consultations

When do your consultations start? It may be earlier than the moment the patient walks into your consulting room. Many consultations have a prologue or overture which begins at the moment the patient becomes aware that you are ready for them and realises that you are calling them into your room, even if you are not yourself present at that moment.

So how do your patients know when you are ready for them? How do you call them? Do you go to the waiting room and greet them by name, do you call them over a tannoy or telephone, or does the receptionist direct them into your room? If you call them yourself, your voice might communicate enthusiasm, boredom, tiredness or irritation. Some practices have a visual display that lights up with the patient's name – and you will notice the patients in the waiting room visually glued to this, waiting for their name to appear in the lights.

Although some of these ways may be relatively fixed and hard to change, you need to think about the effect they may have on the patient at the beginning of the consultation.

- The patient with poor hearing may have been straining to listen out for their name and been really worried about missing their turn. If you are running late, they may have been worrying like this for the last 20 minutes or half hour. That's a lot of time spent worrying.
- Someone with poor sight may struggle to read the illuminated display that tells them where to go.
- If the patient is directed (whether by a disembodied voice over the tannoy or a receptionist) to 'Room 4', do they know where it is? Are they worried they will get lost and walk into the wrong room?
- If your room is a long way down the corridor, the patient with breathlessness or mobility problems may struggle to get to it in good enough shape for the consultation to begin. Think about the last time you ran up half a dozen flights of stairs as fast as possible – it's really hard to give an articulate account of your symptoms if you are fighting to get your breath back as well.
- If the clinician that the patient is consulting either calls the patient over the tannoy or personally collects them from the waiting room, then something about the clinician's mood or state of mind may well come over in this brief, preliminary interaction.

Worry about missing their turn, walking into the wrong room or getting lost can all raise patient anxiety at the beginning of the consultation. As we will discuss later, some patients (and some health professionals too) are not all that good at recognising their emotions for what they are and can filter and distort anxiety so that it emerges as anger, irritation or some other potentially unhelpful emotion.

If you are able to go to the waiting room to collect the patient, the actual consultation starts as you say their name and watch them stand up and walk with you to your room. Use this opportunity to gather more information just by noticing how they look up, stand up and walk.

Beginning the consultation in your room

When the patient gets to your room, what do you say? Think for a moment about your usual opening phrase.

I recently asked a group of doctors to write down the words they use to start their consultations and, although many of them are variations on a theme, I was surprised by the number and variety of different words:

> 'How do you do?'
> 'How are you today?'
> 'Hello, come in. Have a seat.'
> 'Hello, how are you? Come and have a seat.'
> 'Hello, come and sit down.'
> 'Actually that's my chair – this one is yours!'
> 'What can I do for you?'
> 'How can I help you?'
> 'How I can help you?'
> 'Hi – I'm Dr xxxxxxx. I don't think we've met?'
> 'Hello – my name is Dr xxxxxx.'
> 'Good morning/evening.'
> 'That's a nice shirt – where did you get it?' (my all-time favourite for originality and creativity, although I suspect it would wrong-foot most patients).

Many doctors start with a bland, polite, well-meant, helpful question and clearly the commonest ones are variants on 'How can I help you?', 'What can I do for you?' or 'How are you today?'. Of course, there's nothing actually wrong with that, but even these 'neutral' phrases can crowd the patient's first thoughts. An even more effective way to start consultations is to let the patient have complete control. Let's think about this for a moment.

Take a minute or so to recall the most recent time when you yourself were about to be a patient in a consultation – preferably when you were unsure about what was wrong with you and slightly anxious about what was coming next. Think about and recall what it was like being in the waiting room and sitting there waiting to be called in. Try and get a really strong image – remember what you saw, who else was there, what you noticed going on, what the sounds were (for example, radio, music, voices calling patients) and remember the feelings as well. What was going through your mind? Perhaps you were:

- thinking about your symptoms
- getting the sequence of events right
- wondering if you would be able to say everything you needed to say

- experiencing anxiety or even fear about what might be wrong
- worrying about what the doctor will think about you
- feeling anxious about the whole situation of being a patient at all.

You may well have rehearsed in your head the first few words that you would say. Neighbour describes this as a 'gambit' – like the set-piece opening moves of chess that are recognised by all players.

> 'Well I'm no better ...'
> 'I hope I'm not wasting your time but ...'
> 'It's these headaches you see ...'
> 'I've had this sore throat for nearly two weeks.'
> 'I've just come for my Pill.'
> 'I think I'm pregnant.'
> 'I'd like a referral, please.'
> 'I was wondering if you would check my thyroid function.'
> 'I went for an X-ray/blood test/scan – the receptionist said you had the results.'
> 'I wouldn't have come, only I'm going on holiday tomorrow.'
> 'OK – actually there were two things.'

Most patients come into the room with something with which to open the consultation (like the small balloon in Byrne and Long's analogy). They know how they are going to start and they have a good idea what else they want to say, given the chance.

However, sometimes these phrases get overtaken by a spontaneous remark that the patient makes on coming into the room – something they hadn't planned to say, but which is a real eye-opener and may lift the curtain onto their inner world.

> 'Chelsea! Come and sit here *now* – I don't know what I'm going to do with her, I'm at the end of my tether.' (young, harassed-looking mum with a lively toddler in tow)

> 'I thought I was going to have to wait for ever. Don't you realise how busy I am? My time is very valuable you know.' (red-faced, over-weight business man in a striped suit who had been called in because his medication check is well overdue)

> 'Oh, I thought I was seeing Dr Brown. He knows ALL about me.' (middle-aged lady with extensive notes about recent consultations on minor matters)

> 'I'm sorry [in tears], I didn't mean to do this ... those children ... errm ... I mean, they were only playing in the waiting room ... have you got a tissue? I am sorry about this ... I guess ... those children have really upset me.' (female patient, aged 41, childless and with fertility problems)

The doctor who starts their consultation with 'How can I help?', 'What can I do for you?' or 'How are you today?' may well miss the opportunity for the curtain-raising phrase and can also wrong-foot the patient who had already prepared and rehearsed what they were going to say.

Of course some patients, particularly those who know you quite well, will completely ignore the content of your opening phrase, bypass any meaning and hear it simply as 'permission to start talking' – which is probably what you intended anyway! But others will actually respond to what you say. So if you start with 'How can I help you?' or 'What can I do for you?', the patient may actually reply to the question and you might get a response such as:

> 'Er – well I thought I might need antibiotics.'
> 'How can you help me ... well I don't really know. I mean I'm not sure if anyone can help me ...'
> 'What can you do for me? Well, nothing, probably.'
> 'I haven't a clue – that's why I'm here!'

... not necessarily the easiest way for the consultation to start!

Saying almost nothing

If you usually start your consultations with a set phrase, you could try experimenting with saying almost nothing. Clearly, this does not mean sitting and staring at the patient in non-verbal, as well as verbal, silence. If you don't use words, you need to use plenty of non-verbal encouraging gestures and signs, for example smiling, nodding, making eye contact. Try just engaging the patient like this instead of using words, let them start talking and see where you go. Remember, this is not passive behaviour – it needs to be a very conscious, active process on your part with maximum listening and minimum words or interruptions of any sort.

If you are willing to really focus on the patient in the early moments of the consultation, it can pay dividends. You could also think about using words, but without turning them into a question. For example:

> 'Hello, nice to see you. Come and sit down.', followed by non-verbal encouragement.
> 'Hello, Mrs Brown. Come and take a seat.'
> 'Hello there – in you come – sorry you've had to wait.'

The patient can then start anywhere and begin to tell you their story; they don't have to pause and think about how to respond to your question, because there wasn't one. If they have prepared some opening words, they will be able to hold onto these whilst you are saying your own initial greeting.

Example – a cautionary note

Sometimes, changing the way you begin consultations has unexpected consequences. One of my colleagues, a distinguished and popular local doctor, tried beginning his consultations with silence, after going on a course. He was rewarded with a succession of patients who were completely thrown by this behaviour, which was very different from normal, and asked him instead how he was, and whether he was, in fact, ill today!

When you need to say something

There are just a few types of consultations where it is probably better not to use empathic silence with lots of non-verbal encouragers as an opener.

- When the patient has come back at your request because you needed to review them, for the results of an investigation or to discuss a hospital letter. Here silence can easily be misinterpreted as a signal that you have forgotten what this is about. So you could try a pleasantry such as 'Nice to see you again', 'Hello again', followed by:
  - an open question like 'How are you getting on?' and/or
  - a statement used as a question such as 'Now I think you may have come about your test results.'

These openings will let patients get going without you actually imposing an agenda on them. The patient may well be due to come back for test results but actually have come today with something quite different.

- Teenagers can sometimes win at 'staredown' no matter how non-verbally empathic you are being in your attempts to engage them. If you find yourself nodding and saying nothing for very long you might have a consultation that never gets started! Useful phrases in these circumstances might be:

  'It can be difficult to start, sometimes...'
  'Tell me a bit about why you've come today...'.

Doctor-cues

When we think and talk about 'cues' we generally mean those made by patients. But doctors and nurses also give off cues and those at the beginning of the consultation can dictate the whole course of the consultation. Watching videotaped consultations is a good way to pick these up. In the first few moments you can give all sorts of messages to patients, often subconsciously:

  'Oh no, not you again!'
  'I'm in a hurry this morning – let's just have the one problem please and make it snappy.'
  'Ah good – he's come back!'
  'I've got all the time you need today.'

When the patient starts talking

So once the patient has started talking and is clearly in their stride, what do you do? They're in full flow and talking away – when are they going to stop? Do you need to get a word in? Do you interrupt the patient's story or just let them carry on until they've finished? Doctors (particularly) who are in hurry, running late or trying to use limited time efficiently sometimes try to find information quickly by stopping the patient as soon as they have a good idea what's going on and then asking questions. This is, of course, a familiar consulting style in hospital medicine and clinics – the classic way of taking a medical history.

  Patient: er, well, I've got this chest pain ...
  Doctor: Aha! Chest pain. Where is it/what is the character of the pain/does it come and go/does anything make it better or worse/any family history of heart disease/do you smoke/have you had your cholesterol checked? ...

Obviously this is an extreme example, but I have seen many consultation videos of GPs who do consult like this to a greater or lesser extent. One difficulty with this style is that it is very inefficient and you may use up a lot of time going down blind alleys. Far from being a way of getting quickly to the point, it's actually a way of going all round the houses before you do, if ever, get there. The difficulty is this: many patients are not all that good at coming quickly and succinctly to the point or even letting you know why they've (really) come at all until quite late in the consultation. If you start asking them questions, they will, like most of us are taught to do as children, start answering them. They will assume that it's a relevant question because you've asked it and you're the doctor or nurse. So they will try and be helpful and give you the information that they think you want to know. Trying to be efficient and taking hold of the first thing the patient says may well lead to you using up 10 minutes before they say (if they ever do): 'Of course, what I'm really here about is ...'.

Many doctors learnt this style of interrupting patients when they were harassed, overstretched junior hospital doctors. Some persist with it out of the irrational but real fear that patients will carry on talking forever if you let them and never get to the point at all. But patients who are allowed to carry on talking until they stop usually do so after about 2–2½ minutes and by this time they have usually told the doctor almost everything that is relevant.

So, if you are a natural interrupter, why not experiment with letting patients talk until they've stopped? If you feel anxious about this, you could try:

- booking yourself a surgery with a few gaps in it
- booking patients at slightly longer consultation intervals than usual
- doing this on a quiet day when you aren't in a hurry to be finished or to get away to somewhere else.

For this surgery, let each patient talk until they've come to a natural stop. At the first few pauses, try a neutral phrase such as 'I see' or 'Go on', or simply repeat back to them the last few words that they have said to you. Let them keep talking until they really have dried up.

When they come to a real full stop, ask yourself how much information you have already obtained before you have asked even a single question. You may have very little left to ask! You may well find that you already know:

- the symptoms
- the patient's worries
- the patient's real, deep down fears
- what others in the family think
- what they have already tried
- the effect the symptoms are having on home, work, etc
- what they are hoping you might be able to do (if anything).

Doctors who are not used to doing this (for example, GP registrars who have come straight from hospital posts) are sometimes astonished at the efficiency of this method for getting most of the information needed in the consultation in the minimum possible time whilst being very patient-centred. Nurses, in my experience, are generally more skilled than doctors at this.

---

15 minutes that changed the way a group of GP registrars consult

I recently worked with a group of GP registrars at a summer school. Many were sceptical about the benefits of active listening rather than asking questions and so we tried a little exercise together.

I asked them to work in trios – a speaker, a listener and an observer. The 'task' was to find out in maximal detail how one of the others measured a patient's blood pressure, a routine task that all of them had done hundreds of times. I told them that they needed enough detail to exactly match the other person's technique. They had 5 minutes to try each of three different methods, rotating round the three different roles (speaker, listener and observer) each time.

- **Method 1** The listener had to find out information by asking questions and the speaker was asked to answer them fairly minimally with 'yes', 'no', etc.
- **Method 2** The speaker was asked to talk freely about how they measured blood pressure and the listener's role was to listen utterly passively, in silence and with minimal eye contact.
- **Method 3** I asked the listener to ask only open questions, and listen as actively as possible.

The registrars were genuinely surprised to find out how much more quickly they got the information they needed in the third situation, compared with the others. Method 1 was hard work and yielded inadequate information and with method 2, the speaker (who was getting no response) dried up very quickly.

Many of the registrars said this was a revelation that would change the way they listened to patients in the future.

Possible action points

- Watch and listen for the different ways that patients start consultations. Write these down at the end of each consultation. Are they gambits or curtain raisers?
- How do you start consultations? Does it help or hinder the process?
- If you had a complex consultation, what were the early clues? With hindsight, was there something that was apparent from the moment the patient walked through the door? What did you notice?
- Experiment by starting consultations in ways that are different from usual for you. Do these make a difference?
- Video a surgery and watch this either alone or with a colleague, just noticing the beginnings and the first few minutes of the consultation.
    - Who starts the consultation?
    - Gambit or curtain raiser?
    - Do you interrupt?

References and further reading

- Byrne PS, Long BEL. *Doctors Talking to Patients*. London: HMSO; 1976.
- Neighbour R. *The Inner Consultation*. Lancaster: MTP Press; 1987. 2nd edn Oxford: Radcliffe Publishing; 2004.

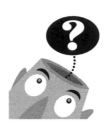

Chapter 4

Building rapport

Key points

- Developing and maintaining rapport are central to effective consulting.
- Rapport means being able to enter a patient's inner world sufficiently to be able to understand it.
- You will find it easier to develop and maintain rapport with some people more than others, but you can (and should) do this with every patient.
- You do not have to like patients in order to develop and maintain rapport with them – just to be willing to enter their world for a short period of time.

Rapport is the ability to be on the same wavelength and to connect mentally and emotionally with others, building mutual trust and respect. In other words, it describes the skills that you need to meet people where they are (wherever that place is). You do not have to like or agree with someone in order to be in rapport, but you do need to know and understand where they are coming from and be willing to meet them there. There is nothing magical about this; although some people find it easier and more natural than others, it is a skill that everyone can learn and that gets better with practice. Good rapport can improve consultations – patients feel listened to, doctors find it easier to understand their patients' problems and outcomes may be better for both the clinician and the patient!

It's worth working hard at developing your skills for building rapport with people. Of course, there will be some patients you like, and then it's quite easy to get into rapport. With other patients, for whatever reason, it may be harder and take longer, but it is still well worth doing.

Recognising and improving rapport

How do you know when you are in rapport with someone? It can be interesting and enlightening to start noticing and observing situations when two people clearly are in rapport and to look at and listen to what's happening. Next time you go to the pub, a restaurant or for a walk in the park, try observing any couple who appear to be getting on quite well with each other. What do you notice? You may see:

- eye contact, i.e. they are looking at each other and into each others' eyes quite a lot of the time
- mirroring of body posture; in other words, they are matching and reflecting each other's physical behaviours, often strikingly so; for example, if one of them has their chin resting on their left hand, the other might mirror this with their own chin resting on their right hand; sometimes, of course, you see even more striking mirroring such as similar clothes and hair cuts!

- lots of simultaneous non-verbal communication (nods, smiles, grunts, etc)
- matching of movements and gestures.

You could also listen to a radio chat show and concentrate on the dialogue between two people. You may hear:

- matching of tone, pace and inflexion
- picking up and using the same words as each other
- descriptions that are visual, auditory or about movement/touching/feeling, and this language matched by the other person.

In consultations you can improve rapport by:

- engaging patients right from the beginning with smiles and eye contact
- a genuine interest and curiosity about the patient and why they are there
- watching and listening for visual, auditory and kinaesthetic (touchy-feely) cues and responding to them (*see* Chapter 5)
- matching the pace and tone of the patient's speech
- matching the patient's language and representational system (visual, auditory or kinaesthetic)
- maintaining awareness of your own body posture and movements (open posture, maintaining eye contact, minimal encouragers)
- matching the patient's body posture
- not interrupting or talking over the patient
- leaving silent space for patients when it is clear that they are thinking hard and 'have gone inside' (eyes looking down and body posture still)
- summarising back to them what they've just said to you to demonstrate that you have listened and understood.

Breaking rapport

As well as knowing how to build rapport, you also need to know how to break it. There are two reasons for this.

- The most important reason is that, if you know what sort of behaviours are used to break rapport, you won't inadvertently and unthinkingly use them at times when it is very important to stay in rapport. A classic example is looking at your watch whilst the patient is in full flow. Only the most insensitive and wrapped-up patient will miss this and most people will stop what they are saying. Another is turning away from the patient to check some detail on the computer screen – it may be well-intentioned, but it's a great rapport-breaker.
- Very, very occasionally, you will find yourself in a consultation where it's not apparent to the patient that time is up and they appear to be ignoring your cues that are saying 'time to leave'. You need to have some tools and skills to help them to recognise this and get out of your room! Here you may need to use rapport-breaking skills. It is, however, very important to use a gradual hierarchy, otherwise the patient may experience you as being abrupt or rude and your relationship with them may be affected.

The tools that break rapport are like a photographic negative of those used to build it. So, just as building rapport is about matching people's speech, behaviour and representational systems, in order to break rapport you need to take active steps to mismatch with the patient. So you might:

- alter your body position so that you are no longer matching that of the patient
- sit up straighter in your chair
- start to speak a little faster and louder than the patient
- break eye contact by looking away
- start to 'play' with the computer
- hand over a prescription, sick note or patient information leaflet
- start to stand up from your chair
- ultimately – walk to the door and open it for the patient.

Possible action points

- Next time you are out and about, or watching a film or listening to the radio, notice when two people are in rapport. What do you observe or hear that tells you this?
- Watch a video of your consultations – either on your own or with a colleague. What are the skills that you use that build rapport?
- Make a conscious effort to build rapport with patients you don't normally like very much by using some of the skills described in this chapter. Does their world look different to you when you do this?
- Practise gently breaking rapport with patients who are reluctant to leave the room.

Further reading

- O'Connor J, McDermott I. *Principles of NLP*. London: Thorsons; 1996.

Chapter 5

Speaking the patient's language

Look with feeling eyes, feel with looking hand

Goethe

Look with thine ears

King Lear, Shakespeare

Key points

- Each of us has a preferred way to take in and process information about the world.
- It's worth working out your own preferred method – visual, auditory, kinaesthetic, or a combination of these.
- Once you know how you are wired up, it is easier to work out your patients' wiring.
- Language content and eye movements can give you clues to help work out what's going on.
- Matching language with patients' helps communication and enhances rapport.
- Scary words (medical jargon, acronyms and long drug names) tend to reduce effective communication. If they have to be used for some reason, teach them to the patient first and check they understand them.

This chapter isn't about communicating in other languages, but about how you can identify and use the patient's preferred way of communicating to enhance your consultations with them. There are three parts to this:

- determining how a patient processes information and using this to find the best way to communicate with them
- listening for and using the patient's own vocabulary of nouns, verbs and adjectives – in other words, speaking the patient's health dialect
- selecting words that are clear and straightforward to understand and ensuring you don't unwittingly use scary words.

The way a patient takes in and processes information

How can you find out how the patient takes in and processes information about the world and their experiences? Unsurprisingly, we don't all do this in the same way! Before you can start to work out how other people do it, it is helpful to have a good idea about how you do this yourself. Even if you think you already know, take a few minutes to reassess and evaluate this.

Many people have two modalities that they work in more or less simultaneously – for example, I know that my preferred methods are auditory and kinaesthetic, and I am much less strongly visual. So it's easy for me to remember the intricate detail of what patients have told me about themselves months ago, including bizarre and probably irrelevant details such as the name of their cat, and I rely on my feelings to help me in the process of the consultation, but I have trouble recognising people, especially out of context. What I've had to learn to do is 'read' people's verbal and non-verbal cues as rapidly as possible, so that I can confabulate long enough to pick up the identifying clues about who they are!

So how do you experience the world?

There are several different ways to work out how you are wired up. First, think about some time recently when you had a memorable day out in a large city, perhaps a shopping trip, city break or somewhere you visited on holiday. What do you remember most clearly? What really stands out now for you? Is it:

- the sight of the buildings, neon lights, traffic whizzing past, colours of the buses, famous sights?
- the sound of the traffic, music from street musicians, conversations that you had or overheard?
- the exquisite tastes of that fantastic meal out?
- the feel of the pavements under your feet, the warmth of the sun (or coldness of rain on your skin), or the emotional feelings such as excitement or anxiety?
- the smell of the city – traffic fumes, food smells from street markets or vendors, exotic spices perhaps?

Try another one. How do you remember phone numbers that you don't already know but need to retain (at least for a short time) and can't write down for whatever reason?

- Do you picture the sequence of numbers as if they were written down? (visual)
- Are you someone who hears the numbers being said out loud or the sequence of sounds that a digital phone makes when you are dialling the number? (auditory)
- Do you remember the pattern that your fingers tap out on the phone keypad (for example, start in the middle, up one, across one, down 2, diagonal)? (kinaesthetic)

Some people use a combination of two of these. Being auditory/kinaesthetic, I say the numbers in my head at the same time as physically moving my finger to the right places on an imaginary standard keypad.

Thinking about people you have met once or twice:

- are you good at recognising them when you see them? (visual)
- would you have trouble recognising them, but instead identify their voice on the phone easily or remember the things they said when you first met? (auditory)

Now try this. Imagine it's one of those busy mornings and you were in a bit of a rush when you left home. In the car driving to work, you have a sudden panic about whether or not you locked the front door behind you. The house key is in your pocket and you're pretty sure you must have locked it because you always do. So how do you recall whether or not you did today:

- by picturing the door and your hand turning the lock or trying the handle (visual)
- by hearing in your head the sound of the key turning (auditory)

- by remembering the feel of the key in your hand and the clunking sensation as the lock turned (kinaesthetic).

Finally, ask yourself these questions:

- what is your name?
- how do you know?

The answer to the first question is obvious, but the second one may cause you to think. Some people know what their name is because they can see it written down, for example over their consulting room door or on a cheque book or letter. Others know their name because they can hear someone calling or saying it. People who are kinaesthetic often find that they just 'know' because it feels right.

So which sort of information do you pick up most easily? Are you primarily visual, auditory or kinaesthetic, or a combination? It's likely that the way you use words and phrases to describe things will reflect your preferred method of processing information and the same applies, of course, to patients.

Visual people

People who are primarily visual (and more people are visual than auditory or kinaesthetic) take in information through what they see. They are often neatly dressed and tend to work in a tidy environment. They find it relatively easy to picture the future and are often good planners. When they talk, they are likely to be able to paint pictures with their words and may include a lot of visual commentary in what they say.

Visual words and phrases include:

'see', 'show', 'reveal', 'colourful', 'appear', 'clear'
'I see what you mean.'
'It's like a black hole.'
'The future looks bleak.'
'I just don't see eye to eye with him.'
'The clouds are lifting.'
'It colours my judgement.'

Auditory people

People who are more auditory take in most information through words and language and from conversations with themselves or with others. They are less concerned than visual people about the state of their immediate local environment – if they live with someone who is visual they may find it puzzling that the visual person cares about the tidiness of the house because they are not so bothered about it.

They often have internal conversations with themselves that can be either helpful or unhelpful. For example:

'You did that well.'
'That was kind.'
'Need to be careful here.'
'Hang on a minute.'

Auditory words and phrases include:

'hear', 'talk', 'sound', 'tell', 'call', 'listen', 'ring'
'That sounds awful.'
'It doesn't ring a bell.'
'He said to me ...'
'I read this article in the local newspaper that said ...'
'I realised that what they were saying on the radio sounded just like me.'

Auditory patients are relatively easy to identify in consultations because they tend to describe the course of their illness and symptoms through describing a conversation they have had with someone else, usually a partner at home, for example:

'... so I said to my husband – "ooh, I felt right queer then" and he said to me "well, you want to get yourself down to the doctor's then", and I said to him, "well, I'll give them a ring tomorrow".'

Kinaesthetic (touchy-feely and doing)

Kinaesthetic people rely on their 'guts' a lot. They take in information through their feelings, both emotional and physical. These people tend to be conscious of their body movements and can often 'feel their way' to an unfamiliar place. They can also enter rooms or buildings and pick up feelings about the environment. Kinaesthetic men often use sporting language or words that describe physical contacts and actions, like 'tackle', 'hold', 'kick', 'grasp', 'run', 'toss', 'step', 'pounce'.

Kinaesthetic words include:
'feel', 'touch', 'hard', 'contact', 'firm', 'grasp', 'soft'
'I can't stand it any longer.'
'I've just got a feeling that ...'
'I just can't seem to grasp that.'
'I've been worried sick.'
'My guts tell me that ...'
'I must tackle this.'
'I just can't get hold of it.'
'It slipped through my fingers.'
'I don't know why! It just feels right!'

Example – visual, auditory or kinaesthetic?

Three people have each been out for a test drive in a flashy new car they might (or might not) want to buy and they are each describing their experience to a friend. The visual one says:

'It's really <u>eye-catching</u> – <u>bright red</u> with seven-spoke alloys and a sun roof. The salesman <u>showed</u> me all the gadgets. Great <u>visibility</u> front and rear. And all those admiring <u>looks</u> I got! I can really <u>see</u> myself driving this car!'

The auditory person says:

'The <u>sound</u> of that engine when you turn the key – a really <u>deep note</u> just like that fantastic <u>throaty sound</u> you get from a TVR. The salesman <u>told</u> me about its ownership history. I really feel <u>in tune</u> with this car. I'll just need to <u>talk</u> it over with my partner before definitely deciding.'

The third says:

'It just <u>felt</u> great! I <u>sank</u> into those leather seats – they really <u>hug</u> you and give fantastic <u>support</u> for your back. And the <u>feel</u> of the wind in my hair when the top was down! When you <u>put your foot down</u> it just <u>kicks</u> you in the back. Mind you, that salesman tried to <u>push</u> me into a decision right there and then. I guess I'll <u>contact</u> him tomorrow – or not!'

The same car – three very different ways of describing the experience.

Understanding eye movements

If you're not sure from their use of language, you can sometimes pick up more clues by watching a patient's eye movements. Each of us stores information in particular places and we retrieve this by looking for it with our eyes, making tiny brief eye movements. There is remarkable consistency across the human race in terms of where we store and retrieve information. It is similar for most people on the planet from almost all ethnic groups, the one exception being people of Basque origin, who for some reason apparently store information quite differently from everyone else.

Visual images

For most people, visual information such as pictures, patterns and images tends to be stored in a plane that is somewhere above eye level. If you notice a patient's eyes flick upwards, it can be worth asking them a 'visual' question, for example:

'How does that look?'
'What were you picturing just now?'
'Tell me what you're imagining.'

There are two different sorts of images – those that we have seen before and therefore remember and those that we have never seen but can imagine. Pictures that are remembered tend to be stored on the opposite side from those that are imagined or constructed. The most common pattern is:

- visual remembered/recalled – eyes flick up and to the patient's left (your right, as you are looking at the patient)
- visual constructed/imagined – eyes flick up and to the patient's right (your left).

So people whose tiny eye movements tend to be upwards may well be primarily visual. If you ask them how they feel about something or what sensations they have, then you may find that their eyes flick up first because they have to conjure up the picture before they can get to the feeling that accompanied it.

Auditory material

Things we have heard and conversations that we have had with others, or that we anticipate having, tend to be stored in the same horizontal plane as the eyes – left or right, but neither up nor down.

As with visual images, auditory experiences that have actually happened and are remembered are stored differently from those that we anticipate, imagine or make up. Generally, sounds that we recall are stored on the left and those that we imagine on the right.

So if a patient's eyes flick horizontally and to the left, you might guess that they are recalling a conversation or something that they have heard. You might ask:

> 'Tell me what was said.'
> 'How does it sound?'
> 'What are you hearing?'
> 'Did you talk to someone about this?'

Sometimes it can be relatively easy to guess what they are internally hearing, so you might say to a female patient whose eyes have just flicked across to the left and whose husband, although not physically present in the consultation, has already had quite a significant voice: 'What did your husband say to that?'

So people whose tiny eye movements are mostly left and right, rather than up or down, are more likely to be auditory than visual.

If you ask auditory people to describe how something looked, they may well first go to the remembered conversation or sound that was going on and then create the picture that you have asked for (eye movements left, then up).

Feelings

The third storage place is for emotions and things that we touch, feel or actively do. These memories tend to be stored downwards and often to the patient's right. So the patient who is looking down and to the right may be recalling something they have touched or a particular emotion. You could ask:

> 'How does that feel?'
> 'How do you feel now?'
> 'What did you feel then?'

The remaining 'storage place' is eyes down and to the left. This place tends to be reserved for internal conversations and you might say:

> 'Tell me what you were saying to yourself just now.'
> 'What did you say to yourself at the time?'

This is summarised in Table 5.1 and Figure 5.1 (but remember that not all patients have read the books and sometimes left and right are interchanged).

It is relatively easy to work out (or 'calibrate' to use a jargon word) where people store information by noticing their eye movements as they say different things to you. So if you ask a patient to describe something that you know they

Table 5.1 Eye movements

	Up	Across	Down
Patient's left	Visual remembered	Auditory remembered	Internal conversation
Patient's right	Visual imagined	Auditory imagined	Kinaesthetic

have already seen, you will be able to observe whether they retrieve this information from their left (more usual) or right (less usual) side.

Matching patients' representational systems is an important tool both to develop rapport and so that patients recognise that you understand or are trying to understand them. If a patient says to you:

'I feel it in my bones.' and you answer 'I see what you mean.'
'The future looks bleak.' and you answer 'It feels like there's no way out.'
'I said to myself, "you really must talk to him about this".' and you answer 'When you thought about that, how did it look?'

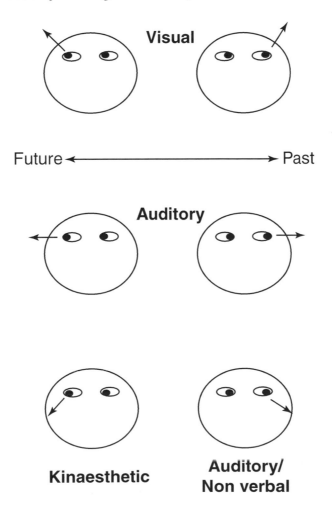

Figure 5.1 A summary of eye movements

they will struggle to connect with your words. They may describe the same actions, thoughts or feelings, but they are in completely different representational systems.

- The patient who 'feels it in her bones' will not have any picture to see.
- The patient who is looking at a bleak future is unlikely to be kinaesthetically feeling a way through it.
- The patient who is having internal conversations with herself is not at all likely to be able to paint a picture to look at.

You may think you've been empathic, but the patient may well feel misunderstood and as if you haven't been listening properly. At best, they will have to pause and tune in to you – rather than the other way round.

Matching the patient's language will mean that you are talking the same 'dialect' as they are. Patients will unconsciously feel that you are in tune with them. Rapport will be improved and there is a good chance that your consultations will go better.

Matching the patient's language

The second aspect of speaking the patient's language is to use their own vocabulary of nouns and verbs. Most patients haven't read the medical textbooks and the words they use to describe their experience of illness or distress are often colloquial or unspecific. The patient with 'tummy pain' may be describing anywhere from the top to the bottom of their abdomen, related to any organ that might be contained in the abdominal cavity and quite a few that aren't! Other patients will try to use medical language perhaps in the hope that this will enable the clinician to tune in better with them. Some patients, particularly those with a keen interest in their health or who are expert patients, may well use medical words with complete accuracy. But others will use words either incorrectly or with only a partially correct understanding. It may be worth exploring this with patients before you take their words at face value.

Clearly, when you are working out what a patient is describing and what's going wrong for them, you will need to clarify at least in your own mind what is going on and which part of the anatomy they are referring to. During this process, you can also learn the patient's dialect for their body parts and functions. When patients use nouns or verbs of their own or dialect words, it is essential to clarify for yourself just what they mean by these before you can move further into the consultation.

Summarising, explaining and planning will be much more effective if you take care to match the patient's language, using their own nouns and verbs. You may be able to introduce more precise language at this point, but make sure that you always link it clearly to the patient's own words.

Example

The patient describing 'tummy pain' was actually experiencing pain in the left iliac fossa and the consulting doctor thought that it was constipation.

> **Doctor A:** OK – this colicky pain that you're getting is coming from your large bowel …
>
> The patient was struggling a bit with exactly what 'colicky' might mean and whether this fitted the tummy pain that she had been getting, so when the doctor said 'bowel' she knew that he was on the wrong lines.
>
> **Patient:** No doctor – it's not in my bowels, it's in my tummy.
>
> As you can imagine, Doctor A was not all that pleased to be interrupted and the consultation risked degenerating into an unhelpful 'tis/'tisn't argument. Doctor B, on the other hand, said:
>
> > OK – can I just check I've got this right? You've been getting tummy pain for a week. It's down at the bottom and more on the left-hand side. Pain in this part of the tummy tends to come from the last part of your gut, which is called the large bowel. I think what's happening is that your large bowel is working more slowly than usual and giving you pain.
>
> The patient was able to clearly hear that Doctor B had understood what she had been saying. She was also educated about anatomy without being in the least patronised. This was quicker, more efficient and avoided any possible confrontation.

Avoiding scary words

The third way to enhance language in consultations is to use words that are safe rather than scary. Doctors and nurses tend to have at least a **B**achelor's degree in **sc**ary words (isn't that what **BSc** or **BS** stands for?) – after all, this is what we are taught at medical school or on nursing courses. Our knowledge and use of this language is one of the key distinguishing features that helps to define us as belonging to the tribe that is 'doctors and nurses' rather than that other tribe – 'patients'. There are three categories of scary words that health professionals use.

Precise language

Sometimes we need precision words in order to communicate accurately with other clinicians, for example 'superior', 'inferior', 'lateral', 'medial', 'radial nerve', 'hypothalamus', 'parathyroid gland' all fall into this category. There are also words that give us short cuts to illness and pathology that we all recognise – 'dissecting aneurysm', 'tension pneumothorax', 'bipolar affective disorder', 'type 1 diabetes' are all short phrases that convey a wealth of information between health professionals.

Drug names

Many drug names are as difficult and unpronounceable as any dinosaur's Latin name, for example bendroflumethiazide, paroxetine, co-fluampicil. No wonder patients get them wrong or use the trade name that happened to be on the latest box: 'No doctor, I don't want that paratoxine, I want my usual Seroxat.'

Acronyms

Health professionals use acronyms all the time when talking with each other – partly as short cuts but, I suspect, mostly as part of the exclusive and excluding code language of our 'tribe'. So is your patient suffering from an acronym? A PE, or an MI, or a raised BP or MS or SLE? Perhaps they are – but the problem is that when any of us meets an acronym that we don't recognise, we spend several seconds internally searching (trawling around inside our heads), trying to work out whether or not we've heard this one before. With the realisation that we don't know this one, there are then several more seconds of trying to guess what the letters might stand for, as well as trying not to look as if we are completely ignorant. Whilst this is going on, it is completely impossible to take in, let alone understand, what the other person is continuing to say. You will notice this sometimes at educational meetings or talks or when listening to a TV or radio show when the 'expert' assumes that everyone else understands the abbreviated short cuts they are using.

In the consultation, there are several possible outcomes:

- the patient completely fails to hear something significant that you say
- they may not like to ask you to repeat it and if you say 'is that OK, everything clear?', they may just nod and agree even though it isn't clear at all
- they may ask you to go over it all again – a poor use of their time and yours
- they may partially hear what you were saying, but misinterpret your meaning.

As seen on video ...

'I need you to get your U and Es checked. And whilst we're at it, let's do a CRP and LFTs ... and, oh yes, we'll get a GGT done too – the lab don't do that unless we've specifically asked for it!'
'I think you've had a TIA.'
'Of course, you had an MI in 1987, so we need to make sure the HDL/LDL ratio is OK.'
'I see you had a CABG done a few years ago.'

Acronyms are generally unhelpful in the consultation and should definitely be avoided altogether if the patient hasn't used them first. Even if they have, it's worth making sure that both you and they think the acronym stands for the same words. The doctor–patient relationship was not exactly enhanced when the doctor wrote 'URTI' on a patient's sick note and the patient interpreted it as meaning 'You are too idle' rather than 'upper respiratory tract infection'.

There's no getting away from these words

Of course there are some words that you sometimes need to use but that, understandably, are very frightening to patients. Words such as cancer, meningitis, heart attack, septicaemia, stroke, pre-eclampsia can hit patients like a punch in the stomach. They can be shocked, winded, dazed and totally blank out anything else that you say whilst they try to get themselves back together. They can be so stunned that they take in absolutely nothing else. Small wonder that patients can come back from the hospital genuinely believing and telling you what they have experienced – that no one told them anything about what would happen next (or at least that they were completely unable to hear anything that anyone said to them after they were told the diagnosis).

But there's no need to use these words

Even in very ordinary consultations about routine problems that are self limiting or treatable, some doctors use words that are unnecessarily scary and worry patients needlessly.

> 'You're dyspnoeic because of mild heart failure, which has caused pulmonary oedema and I'm going to prescribe you some diuretics.'

The patient on the receiving end of this was probably so busy trying to work out the meaning of the words that she missed the treatment plan altogether. The juxtaposition of the words 'failure' and 'heart' was particularly terrifying. When the doctor called the treatment 'water tablets', the patient was really quite puzzled because the problem was with her breathing and there was nothing wrong with her water, thank you very much ... She did start taking the tablets (because the 'apostolic' doctor said so), but they made her run to the toilet all the time which was a real nuisance as she couldn't go out shopping or to see her friends, so she stopped taking them.

This doctor could just as easily have said:

> 'You're a bit breathless because your heart isn't pumping as well as usual at the moment, so some salty water is gathering in your lungs. We need to give you something to get rid of the water and salt, so that your heart has less work to do. You may pass a bit more urine than usual – this is a good sign that the tablets are working for you – and your breathing should be much better soon. Does that make sense?'

This doctor then checked that she had understood and reinforced the message by getting her to repeat it back.

> 'Just so that I know that I've been clear, can I ask you to tell me what you might say to your husband about what you're going to be doing and why?'

And this patient was able to understand what was wrong and why the doctor was prescribing some tablets to help get rid of fluid. Because it made sense to her, she was also more likely to comply.

Sometimes you need to use medical words because there just aren't any others with the same meaning but, in the same way as if you were a language teacher, you can teach these words to the patient first so that they understand what you are talking about and aren't thrown or confused by words they've never heard before.

> **Example**
>
> Have you ever noticed how shocked a patient looks when you tell them they have pityriasis rosea? If you tell them the diagnosis first and then start explaining that it's self-limiting and not 'catching', they can still leave the consultation looking shell-shocked. Here is another way to do it:
>
> > 'I know this rash has worried you, but I can tell you that it is going to get better very soon, whatever we do – even if we do absolutely nothing. It has a long name, which I'll write down for you in a moment in case you want to read up about it or check on the Internet. Here it is – pityriasis rosea. The first word happens to be Greek and it means 'bran' which describes the slight scaliness of the rash – like flakes of bran. The second word just means pink.'
>
> This totally demystifies an otherwise difficult, scary word. It's hard to carry on being anxious about pink bran flakes! This doctor also made sure that the patient already knew that the rash would get better and wasn't anything horrible before they launched into the difficult words.

Table 5.2 lists some examples of words that doctors use (inadvertently) and some less scary alternatives.

Table 5.2 Alternatives for scary words

trauma	cut, bruise, break, etc
deformed	slightly out of shape
examine	look at, feel, listen to
lesion	spot, etc
chronic	persistent
cardiac	heart
failure	not working so well
self-limiting	get better on its own
prognosis	what's likely to happen

Possible action points

Looking at videos of consultations is an excellent way to slow down the process so that you can really notice what is going on. Watch a video of one of your consultations and notice the following points.

- Do you tend to use visual, auditory or kinaesthetic words?
- Can you work out from the patient's language what their preferred representational system is?
- Do you alter your nouns and verbs to take account of the patient's language? If you are visual, do you tend to use visual words with most or all patients or do you change these to match better with patients who are auditory or kinaesthetic?

- How often do you use acronyms? If you do use them, watch the tape very carefully and see how the patient responds.
- How many scary words did you use and what was their effect on the patient?

In your future consultations, try to:

- work out the patient's representational systems
- match the patient's preferred system, particularly if it is different from yours
- use the patient's own nouns and verbs, even if these are not part of your own normal consultation vocabulary
- think about your use of language and work out and use alternatives to acronyms and scary words
- notice whether all of this has an effect on your consultations.

Further reading

- Bandler R, Grinder J. *Frogs into Princes.* Moab, Utah: Real People Press/Eden Grove Editions; 1979.
- O'Connor J, McDermott I. *Principles of NLP.* London: Thorsons; 1996.
- Walker L. *Consulting with NLP.* Oxford: Radcliffe Medical Press; 2002.

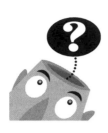

Chapter 6

Managing feelings – your own and the patient's

When in disgrace with Fortune and men's eyes,
I all alone beweep my outcast state,
And trouble deaf Heaven with my bootless cries,
And look upon myself, and curse my fate,
Wishing me like to one more rich in hope,
Featur'd like him, like him with friends possess'd,
Desiring this man's art, and that man's scope,
With what I most enjoy contented least;
Yet in these thoughts myself almost despising,
Haply I think on thee, and then my state,
Like to the lark at break of day arising
From sullen earth, sings hymns at heaven's gate;
For thy sweet love remember'd such wealth brings
That then I scorn to change my state with kings.

Sonnet 29, William Shakespeare

Key points

- Most consultations have an emotional component to them, some more than others.
- Empathy helps the patient to know that you have understood how they felt and why.
- The patient may then feel more satisfied with the consultation.
- Some doctors are reluctant to deal with a patient's emotional issues, but it gets easier to do this with practice.
- Skilled clinicians can use their own feelings in the consultation to help them work out what the patient is feeling – in other words, as an additional diagnostic tool.

The vast majority of consultations in primary care have an emotional component to them, every bit as important as any physical symptoms.

Sometimes, the patient's emotional needs form the core part of the consultation, for example:

- a man of 52 is feeling low, not sleeping, anxious and wondering if life is not worth living
- a woman aged 35 can scarcely leave the house because of panic attacks
- the parents of a 26-year-old who has committed suicide.

In others, there is an emotional component of equal significance to the physical symptoms:

- a woman of 70 has had breast cancer and is getting a severe pain in her back (and is worried sick that she has bony secondaries)
- a six-year-old boy, whose father was killed recently in an accident at work, comes with abdominal pain and nightmares
- a woman of 40 has a black eye and is worried her nose is broken; these injuries were inflicted by her husband at home last night and it wasn't the first time.

Even consultations that appear to be purely about physical symptoms or non-emotional needs are still likely to have emotional undercurrents.

Example

A 45-year-old teacher has come for a renewal of her sick note. She has been off work since she was assaulted by a pupil at school and her shoulder was injured. She has had physiotherapy and anti-inflammatory pain killers, but her shoulder is still very stiff and sore and she isn't able to lift her arm to write on the board. Although this may seem fairly straightforward (and if you are in a hurry it would be an easy consultation to deal with in 2 minutes), there may well be complex underlying emotional factors, such as:

- anger and frustration that it is taking a long time for this to get better
- anxiety because she is now on half pay and this will soon go down even further – the mortgage still needs to be paid
- relief that she no longer has to do a job that was getting increasingly stressful
- fear for the future: Will she work as a teacher again? Can she retrain to do anything else? What about her pension?
- loss of status – she is now 'just a housewife' in her own eyes and those of others
- loss of relationships with her colleagues at school, who were sympathetic at first but are now losing interest
- boredom and frustration at being at home with nothing much to do other than watch the daytime soaps on the television
- relationship difficulties due to changed dynamics with her husband – they used to have an 'equal' partnership, but now it is very unequal
- grief for loss of health, self-esteem and friendships with colleagues.

So how can health professionals deal effectively with patients' emotions? The key tool here is empathy, defined by the Native American Indians as 'walking a mile in another man's moccasins' and by Chambers Dictionary as 'the power of entering into another's personality and imaginatively experiencing his or her experiences'. In other words, being able to be in tune or in touch with another person's feelings and experiences in such a way that you can have some idea of the effect that these are having on their life and their world. Clearly, you can never actually know or feel what it is like for the patient, so the phrase 'I know how you feel' is almost always untrue and may be received as empty and hollow by the patient.

Recognising and acknowledging feelings

At its most basic level, empathy is about recognising a patient's feelings and acknowledging these with words, or non-verbally or both:

- 'You look sad about that.'
- 'You seem very relieved!'
- 'I wondered if you were upset just now.'

At a slightly more sophisticated level, there are three stages in an empathic response:

1. recognising and identifying the emotion that the patient is feeling
2. being able to identify where the feeling has come from, in other words what has happened to the patient to have caused it
3. putting the two together and responding to the patient in such a way that they know that you have made this connection.

There are also two separate components – feeling and thinking (or emotional and cognitive, if you prefer). You need to be able to:

- **feel** in order to recognise the emotions
- **think** so that you can work out where they've come from
- and both **think and feel** so that you can acknowledge these to the patient in a useful and helpful way.

Recognising the feeling

Clearly, the first step is to notice that there is some sort of emotional current running in the consultation. At times this will be obvious, for example when the patient:

- is tearful
- is red in the face, shouting and clearly very angry
- is clearly immensely relieved about test results and is looking joyous and happy.

At other times it is a bit less obvious and may be something that you pick up either from the content or the delivery of what the patient is saying to you.

Content

The patient may vocalise their feelings along these lines:

- 'It's been just awful.'
- 'At times, I don't know how I've been able to go on at all.'
- 'You don't know how afraid I've been.'

Delivery

This is about the patient's non-verbal cues, which, once you've noticed them, you can either explore (at the time or later) or choose to ignore. The cues include:

- facial expressions
- hesitancy, as in 'ums' and 'ers'

- a slight slowing of their speech
- a mismatch or incongruence between the words and the manner of delivery or expression.

Making the connection

Here it is useful to put on the moccasins (metaphorically speaking) and to imagine how you might feel if you, for example:

- had a progressive, debilitating illness
- had just been on the receiving end of bad news
- had recently been bereaved
- were waiting for the results of significant investigations
- had just been told that all the tests were clear.

Responding

You can, of course, respond both verbally and non-verbally. As always, the non-verbal part is very important and few patients will be fooled by the right words with the wrong (or no) feelings attached to them. A robotic response accompanied by boredom, indifference or a complete lack of genuineness is worse than useless.

Sometimes you can get away without using words at all – just sitting in silence with the patient, perhaps leaning forward, touching their arm, or nodding, smiling or making an appropriate gesture.

'Allowing' feelings

Some patients have difficulty in acknowledging or expressing feelings and may need permission. Particular 'at risk' groups here are some men (of an age when a 'stiff upper lip' was considered to be a positive attribute for coping with adversity) and others from families where feelings were regarded as something rather unpleasant or even dangerous, to be suppressed and buried as soon as possible.

It is not always easy to help patients to express their feelings and sometimes this may be a 'consultation' that is spread over weeks, rather than minutes. Some useful tools here are:

- acknowledging that you notice that the patient is feeling something: 'I can see how upset you are about this.'
- my friend John: 'Many people in your position would be quite upset about what's happened. I well remember when a good friend of mine went through something similar and it took a while for him to adjust and get back on his feet – but he did get there in the end.'
- tentative suggestions: '… angry, even'
- explicit permission: 'It's OK to feel sad/angry/relieved.'
- softeners: 'I'm just wondering whether you feel …'.

Self-disclosure

Small doses of self-disclosure may occasionally be helpful, but note the key words here are 'occasionally' and 'small' – it is not helpful to anyone if the consultation becomes a conversation about feelings in adverse circumstances or if the clinician's experiences are allowed to crowd out those of the patient or, at worst, the roles become temporarily reversed in the consultation and the clinician becomes the patient and the patient becomes the listener.

> 'I remember well how sad I felt when my grandmother died, so I'm not at all surprised that you're so upset; she has been an important person for you and I know she has been there for you when you've had problems at home and when it's felt like there wasn't anyone else you could turn to.'

From time to time a clinician can genuinely and completely empathise with the feelings of a patient (for example, if they have also had a depressive illness or have a relative who is dying from cancer). It is particularly important in these circumstances for the clinician to be sufficiently self aware so that they can hold back from letting their own experience and feelings get in the way of the patient's.

Real or 'authentic' feelings

Sometimes a patient's feelings can seem totally bizarre and difficult to understand, for example:

- a middle-aged man with recurrent central chest pain is angry with you
- a woman, whose son has just killed himself, appears totally serene and tells you that it was probably for the best
- a woman, who has just learnt that she does not, after all, have secondaries in her lungs from her breast cancer, is sad.

This seems bizarre and can feel confusing. You might expect the above three patients to be, respectively, anxious, sad and devastated, and relieved.

One of Eric Berne's (1970) really useful concepts is that all of us, as children, learn that there are some feelings that we are allowed to express in our families as we are growing up and others that are not allowed and become taboo. He described four 'authentic' feelings: sadness, happiness, fear and anger.

Most families will 'allow' expression of three of these, but some may have more difficulty with the fourth. If an adult patient appears, for example, angry when you might expect them to be afraid, it might be because 'fear' is a disallowed feeling. In other words, the real feeling has become displaced and substituted by a different one, called a 'racket feeling'. The word 'racket' is used here to mean a dodge or scam, rather than a tennis racket. It's a bit like having a paint box of colours (emotions), but some of the colours are missing. If you had to paint a picture of a daffodil, but didn't have any yellow in your paint box, you might well use a different colour such as red or blue instead.

Example

Henry, a 50-year-old man with chest pain, saw his own father displaying anger in all sorts of situations and witnessed that this was 'rewarded' by other family members paying attention, being afraid and subservient, stroking him and generally rewarding this behaviour. When he was growing up at home, he developed all sorts of different shades of anger (red?) in his emotional palette.

> As a small child he had been afraid of the dark but instead of being treated with compassion and sensitivity, he was instead punished with verbal abuse for expressing this emotion: 'My god. Afraid of the dark. Crying at your age!! What a big girl's blouse you are, lad.'
>
> Understandably, he learnt that fear was prohibited or taboo and so did not develop the ability to express it. (There were no shades of this colour (yellow?) in his emotional paint box.)
>
> As a 50-year-old adult, he cannot express fear to you because it is a disallowed emotion, so instead he displays an emotion that is allowed and that he is very familiar with – anger.

Awareness of this kind of behaviour can help you to understand why a patient might sometimes display feelings that seem quite inappropriate. This helps you to avoid responding in an understandable but unhelpful way to someone's unexpected emotions, such as apparently inexplicable anger with you.

One's own feelings in the consultation

Health professionals are manifestly not robots and also have feelings in the consultation. In my view, Balint's (1957) major contribution to the GP–patient consultation process was in acknowledging and making explicit the fact that the doctor has such feelings, that these can affect the patient and the consultation process, and that the doctor's feelings can be affected by the patient (transference and counter-transference). If the doctor recognises this, then their feelings can increase their understanding of the patient.

This may seem obvious now, but it was a major change in thinking at a time when, generally speaking, 'doctors knew best' and demonstrated their professionalism by an absence of feelings or emotions. At that time, the doctor's feelings were generally considered to be a problem, or weakness, that needed to be concealed from the patient. The medical model of the consultation (patient presents symptoms, doctor makes diagnosis and prescribes treatment, patient goes away) didn't allow for anyone's emotions getting in the way of a 'scientific' process.

Using feelings in a helpful way

There are times in consultations when you will have strong feelings, but know that these have to be kept under wraps because expressing them at the time would be unsafe or interfere with the consultation process. For example in an emergency situation, it would be unhelpful to panic, weep or be inconsolable with grief. But these feelings are real and may well need to be acknowledged and expressed later, perhaps by debriefing with a colleague once the emergency situation is under control and the patient is safe. This sort of emotional off-loading is very important to keep you in good shape and help to avoid blunting of feelings and emotional burnout. Most health professionals have learnt to recognise and acknowledge their feelings but also, generally, to appropriately restrain them within the consultation process, dealing with them later instead.

However, from time to time something about what's going on in the consultation affects us so much that very active feelings come to the surface. For example:

- **sadness** – for example when parents come to tell you that their only, much wanted baby has a rare, incurable, metabolic illness and will die within a year
- **happiness** – shared with a patient when the feared diagnosis is disproved
- **fear** – when a drug user comes into your room and is in no mind to leave until you produce a prescription for him
- **anger** – on hearing a mother's acute distress that her trusted babysitter has been sexually abusing her young daughters.

There are other times when the consultation appears to be mostly about physical symptoms, but you start to become aware of feelings coming to the surface in yourself. Paying attention to these feelings can be very useful diagnostically and can give you a real and unexpected insight into what a patient is feeling. In the jargon, this is called 'counter-transference' – feelings that arise in the health professional as a result of the consultation; in other words, feelings that were not present in the health professional before the patient walked into the consulting room and are likely, therefore, to have arisen from the patient themselves.

Example

Jim is a middle-aged man, who has been unable to work for many years because of fibromyalgia. He comes to see you for his three-monthly sick note and tells you about one symptom, then another, then another. None of the symptoms seems connected and they are all fairly minor, but clearly troubling him (an area of dry skin on his arm, poor sleep pattern, feeling dizzy when he stands up, an ache in his knee).

Asking yourself the question 'How am I [as the clinician] feeling at this moment?' gives you the answer 'wading through treacle, really quite overwhelmed by all of this, struggling to see a way forward and a sense of hopelessness that I can do anything useful to help'.

Recognising that you definitely weren't experiencing any of these feelings before the patient came into the room leads you to realise that these feelings are probably arising from the patient. This is now useful in two different ways.

- It helps to prevent you from believing that these feelings are because of your own incompetence, inexperience or inability: 'If only I were a better doctor/read some more books/went on the right course, then I would know what to do to help Jim'.
- It also gives you a new tool to use because you can reflect how you are feeling back to the patient and this may give them new insights:

  'You've been telling me about your dry skin, dizziness, poor sleep pattern and aching knee and I can understand how difficult you must find all of this. I'm just wondering whether you might be feeling overwhelmed, struggling to find a way forward and even, perhaps, a sense of hopelessness?'

This is a very powerful way of giving insight to patients. You need to choose your moment carefully to use it. In the above example, it is used at the summarising stage of the consultation and the clinician is demonstrating that they have heard enough of the story and been listening well because they are able to repeat and reflect back Jim's symptoms to him. It is also wise to use a 'softener' like 'I'm just wondering' or 'perhaps' as a way of showing that you are tentatively exploring this rather than behaving like a mind-reader. This also then allows the patient to consider what you have said and either accept or reject it. This may be because you are partially or completely wrong: 'Well ... sort of ... actually it's more that I feel so upset that I can't work and provide an income for the family.'

Or it may be that you are right, but the patient is not able to realise or accept this at that moment. Even if, during the consultation, they flatly reject what you are saying, your words may continue to resonate for them after it has finished and you may find that they have, emotionally, moved on a bit by the next consultation.

So, next time you start feeling inexplicably sad, angry, overwhelmed or as if there is no way out, consider whether these feelings belong to the patient and are coming from them, not you.

Transference and counter-transference

Counter-transference, then, is an expression used more frequently by psychologists and counsellors than doctors, but names a process that is very useful to primary care clinicians. It refers to feelings that arise in the clinician but that have come from the patient. Transference, on the other hand, refers to feelings of attachment or affection that the patient develops for the clinician. The psychiatrist Sigmund Freud first described these and the commonly quoted example is of the patient who believes they have fallen in love with their doctor or nurse.

Crying with patients

Just occasionally, there may be situations when you shed tears with a patient, such as a parent whose child has died or the bereaved family you have looked after for some time. No patient that I have ever come across has minded this ultimate expression of empathy.

Helping emotionally upset patients

What do you do when a patient is very upset and perhaps crying in your surgery? Clinicians vary in how comfortable they feel with patients who cry and there are, of course, different ways to respond. There is no absolute right or wrong way to do this and what you actually do will depend on a combination of who the patient is, what your relationship with them is like, the underlying reason for the upset, how you are feeling yourself in that moment and what sort of external pressures you are experiencing (for example, running late, lots of visits, a meeting for which you would prefer not to arrive late).

Clinicians who are particularly uncomfortable when patients cry sometimes abort the crying before it even starts. For example, they change the subject or start to talk to the patient, perhaps slightly raising their voice, either in volume or pitch. This can 'break the state' that the patient is in and prevents the patient from breaking down into tears.

If the patient does start to cry despite the clinician's conscious or unconscious attempts to prevent this happening, then those who are uncomfortable will use words or gestures to stop the crying as soon as possible: 'There, there! No need for that, now! Here, dry your eyes' (passing a tissue).

Other clinicians might let the patient cry, perhaps sitting quietly, leaning forward or moving their chair a little closer to the patient. It is a personal and individual decision whether to touch the patient or not, and most clinicians trust their instincts. Sometimes it can feel right to touch a patient's arm, hold their hand or put an arm around their shoulders. At other times, it doesn't feel right. There are particular situations where you may need to be cautious in order to avoid the danger of misinterpretation – particularly perhaps if you are an older male with a younger and vulnerable female patient (or vice versa).

A box of tissues is essential and something that should always be close by (though perhaps in a drawer rather than on display). There is nothing worse than reaching for the tissues only to find that the last person to use your room has either moved the box to a new place or used the last one and not bothered to replace the box! The timing of handing over the tissues is important – it can be both used by the clinician and interpreted by the patient as a signal to stop crying and move on; so think for a moment before you hand the box over.

The BATHE model

How else can you help patients who are very emotionally distressed? One useful model is given the acronym BATHE. It helps move consultations forward constructively, avoiding both doctor and patient wallowing in the awfulness or hopelessness of the situation. As clinicians, we can sometimes be tempted to offer our own solutions to patients (trying to 'make it better' perhaps). Using this very practical brief psychotherapy model will help you to enable patients to find their own ways forward instead. There are five tight foci to the model:

* **B**ackground
* **A**ffect
* **T**rouble
* **H**andling
* **E**mpathy.

Background

> **Question:** 'What's going on in your life right now?'

This question helps you to understand the patient's situation. The qualifying phrase 'right now' helps the patient focus on the here-and-now rather than launching into an epic saga dating from 1970.

Affect

> **Question:** 'How is this affecting you?' or 'How do you feel about that?'

This moves the patient forward from a description of events, conversations, home, work, etc. It acts as a punctuation mark in their thoughts so that they can tell you more easily what is specifically causing them problems, difficulties or distressing feelings. As with any consultation, you cannot assume or correctly guess what it is that the patient is feeling – you have to ask the question!

Trouble

> **Question:** 'What is troubling you most?'

This is a focusing tool which will help the patient to tell you what it is that is really getting on top of them. The key word is 'most' and the patient's response to the question can lead you to the central problem.

Handling

> **Question:** 'How are you handling this?'

This question has two effects. First, it moves the problem forward again from defining it clearly into talking about actions. It also has an implicit meaning (a presupposition) that the patient *is* handling it. In other words, it shifts responsibility for the problem back to the patient. This is useful for both apparently helpless patients and also for well meaning, but overhelpful, clinicians.

Empathy

> **Statement:** 'I can understand that this must be difficult for you.'

This empathic remark helps to balance the practical nature of the other parts of the model. Equally, it expresses caring and concern without implying that the clinician can make it better or has a solution, or that the patient should hand over responsibility for the problem to the clinician.

Summary

Although this model sounds simplistic, it is based on very effective brief psychotherapeutic techniques. It actively discourages the patient from developing dependency on the doctor (bad for both patient and doctor) and instead helps the patient to explore realistic coping strategies. It is a model that works with and supports the patient's own coping strategies (however embryonic), and encourages further development of coping skills and responsibility for their own behaviours, feelings and actions.

Possible action points

- Watch and listen for the patient's feelings – ask yourself whether they are 'authentic' or 'racket' feelings.
- Which feelings do you find easiest yourself? Is there one of the four authentic feelings that you know you find harder to feel?
- Watch for counter-transference feelings. Do feelings that arise in you seem to be coming from the patient? Can you use this to help you move the consultation forward, perhaps by checking out these feelings with the patient?
- Try out the BATHE model next time you have a distressed or apparently helpless patient.

References and further reading

- Balint M. *The Doctor, his Patient and the Illness.* London: Pitman Medical; 1957. 2nd edn Edinburgh: Churchill Livingstone; 1964, reprinted 1986.
- Berne E. *Games People Play: the psychology of human relationships.* London: Penguin Books Ltd; 1970.
- Jacobs M. *Psychodynamic Counselling in Action.* London: Sage Publications; 1988.
- McCulloch J, Ramesar S, Peterson H. Psychotherapy in primary care – the BATHE technique. *Am Family Physician.* 1998; **57**(9): 2131–4.
- Rogers C. *On Becoming a Person – a therapist's view of psychotherapy.* London: Constable; 1986.

Chapter 7

Getting patients to tell you what's wrong

Under the look of fatigue,
The attack of migraine and the sigh
There is always another story,
There is more than meets the eye

'The Secret is Out', WH Auden*

There's language in her eye, her cheek, her lip;
Nay, her foot speaks

'Troilus and Cressida', William Shakespeare

Key points

- Active listening helps patients to tell their stories to you.
- Asking less and listening more is very time-efficient.
- It is as important to listen for what is not said, as to listen to what is said.
- Sometimes patients would like to tell you things but are restrained by their own internal 'policemen'. It is worth learning to recognise when these policemen are active – and to explore what is being inadvertently concealed.
- Finding out what patients are really worried about is well worth doing. If you make assumptions about these worries, the chances are you will be wrong. You can't effectively advise or reassure patients if you haven't actually found out what they are worrying about.

It may seem obvious. Patients come in, sit down and start talking. They give you a lot of information, you try and make some sense of it, deal with the problems and out they go.

But it's worth taking the trouble to think about how you hear what the patient is really saying to you. This may mean that you need to examine your toolkit of listening skills and start to refine and hone them as well as, perhaps, adding new skills. There will be many skills that you have already and that are part of your own intuitive style of consultation. But there may be others that you could practise and add to your repertoire.

When patients feel as if they have been really listened to, several things can happen:

- they find the consultation more satisfactory
- they are more likely to tell the doctor or nurse what they are really worrying about

---

*Reproduced with permission of Faber and Faber Ltd from *Collected Poems* by WH Auden.

- the relationship between health professional and patient is enhanced by the process of the consultation
- health professionals find the consultation more satisfactory as well!

We have already looked at the importance of developing and maintaining rapport with patients and clearly this is a prerequisite for getting them to tell you what's wrong with them. Few patients can unburden themselves if they don't feel that the clinician in front of them is somewhere on their wavelength!

So what are the key skills that help patients tell their stories? Many of these come under the heading of active listening skills.

Active listening skills

When we watch the television or a film, we listen passively – the narrative goes on and on irrespective of what we do. You can fall asleep or go and make a cup of coffee and that party political broadcast or game show will just carry on regardless. Nothing that you do will make any difference to the speaker – even if you get so bored or fed up that you switch off the television or walk out of the film, they will just carry on to other listeners instead! Clearly this is passive listening.

Active listening means taking an active participative role in the process of another person talking to you. This is different from a conversation where there is normal toing and froing and in which people more or less take turns to contribute to the process. In active listening, one person has the role of talker, and the purpose of the other (the health professional in the consultation) is to enable them to say what they want to say, in their own words, in a way that is as full of meaning as possible to both of them. There are particular skills that enhance active listening: body posture, using encouraging noises and gestures, echoing the patient and asking open questions.

Body posture and how you sit

You need to demonstrate to the patient through your musculoskeletal system, as well as in your words, that you are interested in them and in what they are saying. This will include the following techniques.

- Use a chair that puts you and the patient at the same height, so that you can look at them face to face and neither of you is 'looking down' on the other.
- Sit close enough to be near the patient without actually being on top of them and invading their personal space. There is quite a narrow therapeutic window here. Sit too far away and you can feel distant, too close and you can both feel very uncomfortable. You could borrow a colleague and experiment with each sitting in the consulting doctor's chair and the patient's chair, moving away from each other until you both feel remote, then together again. 'Reach out and touch' is quite a good distance to be apart – not so close that you are on top of each other, but close enough to touch a hand or arm if this is appropriate.
- Face the patient, ideally at an angle of about 45 to 90 degrees. Being faced directly can feel threatening. It also means that you have to make an active effort to look away from the other person. If you sit at 45 degrees, then you can each naturally break eye contact without actually looking as if you are being antisocial or distracted!

- Use eye contact; look at the patient and be attentive to them by nodding and smiling.
- Use an 'open' body posture, with your knees uncrossed, your arms unfolded and sitting up rather than being hunched into a ball.

Encouraging noises and gestures

This is about using a language of sounds rather than words to help patients to continue with the process of telling their stories, once they've started. Encouraging noises include: 'yes ... yes', 'mm ... mm', 'I see', 'go on', '... and then?', 'uh ... hh', 'right', '... and so?', 'ah ha'. These may need to be interspersed with more specific and particular words or phrases such as: 'Now I understand.', 'That sounds dreadful!', 'How awful for you.'

Every health professional will have their own vocabulary of these 'minimal encouragers' and they need to go hand in hand with a set of encouraging gestures such as smiling, nodding and looking interested.

Echoing

Another useful tool is to repeat or echo the patient's last word or few words. This particularly helps patients who are not very fluent in describing their symptoms or are hesitant about what they are telling you. It's tempting to assume that their first phrase or two is all you are likely to get and to start firing questions. When you ask questions, the best you can hope for is answers – but repetition is likely to get you much more information in a shorter length of time.

You need to be in rapport with the patient to do this and then, quite simply, just echo back to them the tail end of what they say to you with a slightly rising inflexion – in other words the pitch of your voice goes from a lower note to a higher note as you say the word(s) so that it has a slight questioning sound to it, for example:

> **Patient:** Err ... I've had this pain in my left arm ... (pause)
> **Doctor:** Left arm?
> **Patient:** Yes – just here (running hand up and down the arm) – it's like a toothache ... (pause)
> **Doctor:** Toothache?
> **Patient:** Yes ... sort of dull and heavy ... and I've had it a bit in my chest as well.
> **Doctor:** In your chest as well?
> **Patient:** erm ... it came on when I was gardening ...
> **Doctor:** When you were gardening, eh?
> **Patient:** Yes – a really heavy pain in my chest that made me sweaty ...
> **Doctor:** Sweaty?
> **Patient:** And quite out of breath too ... (pause)
> **Doctor:** Sweaty and out of breath?
> **Patient:** You don't think it's my heart, doc, do you?

You get the idea. This is a much more efficient way of learning what is wrong with the patient, and what they are worried about, than just firing questions one after another.

Open questions

Open questions are the ones that help open patients up and enable them to tell you more. They are different from closed questions, which are ones that can be answered with 'yes' or 'no', and semi-closed questions, which can be answered with very short (and generally not very helpful) answers.

- **Closed question** 'Have you had chest pain?' (answer: 'yes'/'no')
- **Open question** 'Tell me about your chest pain.' (can't be answered 'yes'/'no')
- **Semi-closed question** 'When did it start?' (answer: 'yesterday' or 'Tuesday'; limited information gained)
- **Closed question** 'Are you depressed?' (answer: 'yes'/'no'/'I don't know')
- **Open question** 'How have you been feeling lately?' (can't be answered 'yes'/'no').

Some particularly useful open questions are:

- 'Tell me more.'
- 'What have you tried?'
- 'In the middle of the night, most people find that their imagination is a bit over active and everything can seem much worse than it perhaps really is ... what's your worst fear in the night about this?'

This last one is especially helpful when you suspect that a patient has fears that they are too embarrassed or uncomfortable to tell you about (such as cancer, sexually transmitted infections, AIDS). It is easier to answer than the more direct and confrontational question: 'What are you worrying about?' It is also easier for the patient than if you ask a closed question, which might feel unintentionally blunt or even off the mark altogether, for example: 'Are you worrying this is cancer/angina/something really serious?' Of course if they really weren't worrying at all about cancer before you asked the question, they certainly will be now. After all, it must be a possibility or you wouldn't have mentioned it, would you?

Closed and semi-closed questions

There is also a place for these in the consultation, but it comes later on. When the patient has said all they need to, there may come a moment when they've dried up and you know most of what's wrong, but there are a few key points that are missing. This is the place to ask closed questions such as:

> 'You've told me a lot about your tummy pain and I just need to ask you one or two more questions first, then I want to examine you' (signposting, i.e. telling the patient what to expect now and soon). 'Does it wake you in the night? Are your bowels just the same as usual or has there been any recent change?'

Or to the patient with sciatica:

> 'There are two important questions that I need to ask you. They may sound a bit strange, but bear with me! Do you have the same urge as normal when you need to pass water? Is there any numbness around your bottom?'

Listening for what's not said

There are two key aspects to this:

- information that you would expect to hear but the patient isn't revealing at the moment – a conscious or semi-conscious withholding
- speech censoring – an unconscious withholding.

Conscious withholding

Sometimes the patient isn't sure whether something is relevant or not. They aren't deliberately withholding – they're just not sure whether or not to say it now, later or not at all. Or it may not even have occurred to them that you might be interested. Asking appropriate open or closed questions is likely to reveal this information fairly readily.

Speech censoring

This is different from conscious withholding and happens when the patient holds something back without realising it. Speech censoring alerts you to the possibility that something of significance to the patient is being unknowingly withheld and can lead you to the really interesting area of the patient's blind spots.

A recent advertisement encouraging us to have more understanding of people with autism said something like:

> 'What's the first thing an autistic person sees when they come into a room? Answer: a stain on the carpet shaped like France, a postcard sticking up from behind an ornament, six cushions with tassels, 28 chair legs, dust on the piano ...'

In order to live in the world and make sense of it, we use powerful filters to sift out far more information than we ever take in. If we didn't, we would be permanently overloaded with information and relatively helpless, just trying to identify the wood from the trees. A powerful censoring engine is at work in each of us all the time. Mostly, this is a very helpful tool that enables us to get on with the process of living, but sometimes it means we are living with outdated beliefs about ourselves or others. There has usually been a good reason for these beliefs developing – perhaps a significant event led to their development. But they may now be holding us back or giving us false or mistaken ideas.

There are three different ways that patients may demonstrate this type of information censoring and they are: generalisations, deletions and distortions.

Generalisations

These are statements that patients make that include strong phrases that are all-encompassing and unlikely to be wholly true. They generally contain the words 'always' or 'never', for example:

> **Patient:** I always need antibiotics.
> **Challenge:** Always? For everything? What might happen if you didn't get antibiotics?

Patient: I never get headaches.
Challenge: This is usually, of course, said when the patient has got or had a headache.
Patient: I'm terrified of hospitals.
Challenge: Which hospitals have you been to? So what happened there that upset you so much?
Patient: But I've always smoked.
Challenge: Really? Well you must have started sometime! That means you can stop as well – if you choose to.

Deletions

Deletions happen when the patient says something and you are really not at all clear what they are referring to. A whole chunk – often a very significant noun or verb – is completely missing, meaning that their statement makes little or no sense, for example:

Patient: They ought to do something.
Challenge: Who are 'they?' What is the 'something' that 'they' ought to do?
Patient: It's no better.
Challenge: What's no better? What is 'it'?

Distortions

Do you remember nouns and verbs from junior school grammar lessons? My own memory of them is that 'nouns are naming words' and 'verbs are doing words'. Nouns tend to have more permanence because they name something that already exists. Verbs permit more change, because they describe actions. Distortions occur when patients use nouns, rather than verbs, to refer to actions. This happens when an action or process has got stuck somewhere (a bit like a flow of water that has become solidified into ice). The implication is that it is now fixed and unchangeable. Let's have a look at a few examples to illustrate this.

Patient: I feel a failure.

'Failure' is a noun, but what the patient is really saying is that they perceive that they have failed (verb). This can then be challenged in different ways:

*   What did you fail at?
*   Do you always fail at everything? Really? Well you were successful at getting an appointment with me today and that's not always easy!
*   Tell me three things where you were successful today.

Patient: It's his attitude.

Again 'attitude' is used here as a noun, but the speaker is really describing behaviour that gives them information about his attitude.

*   What did he do?
*   How can you tell?
*   What would make a difference?

Patient: She is unmanageable.

Here there are two distortions: 'manage' is a verb being used as a 'stuck' noun. But the person who can't 'manage' here is the speaker. You could ask:

- What does she do?
- How do you feel then?
- How does it affect you?
- What strategies could you try?

Challenging deletions, distortions and generalisations

This helps the patient in several ways.

- It takes you closer to the patient's model of the world. The more you understand of their model, the more likely it is that you can help them.
- It challenges unreasonable beliefs that may be limiting them in what they are doing or are able to do.
- It can help to open up new pathways and reframe the situation so that people can see new possibilities for change.
- Like Spring, it can thaw the ice of a noun and reframe it as the flow of a verb.

Cues

During consultations, patients give out signals or cues, which may be in words or non-verbal. These signals can give the clinician keys to really significant information – if only he or she notices them in the first place. Clinicians who are learning to consult can find it hard enough just to hold onto the overt information that the patient is giving them, make a diagnosis and formulate a sensible management plan – cues may be missed.

The ability to recognise cues, to hold onto the recognition until the right moment comes along and then make use of the cue in some helpful way does get easier with practice. In particular, videotaping consultations and then looking at the video is an excellent way of starting to become more aware of cues. Examples of cues and what to do about them are given in Table 7.1.

Table 7.1 Cues and what to do about them

Cue	What it might mean	Examples of what you might say or do	Pitfalls of missing the cue
Both parents come in with a small child when normally just one of them would come.	They are really worried that there is something seriously wrong with the child.	When you have built rapport, found out about the problem and summarised back, ask 'I can see that you are both worried – can you tell me what thoughts you have had yourselves about what might be wrong with ...?'	The parents are not reassured by what you say and may leave still dissatisfied and worried.

Table 7.1 (Continued)

Cue	What it might mean	Examples of what you might say or do	Pitfalls of missing the cue
A patient is accompanied by their husband/ wife/partner when you normally see them alone.	One or both of them is worried about what's wrong. The accompanying partner may be afraid that the patient will not tell you everything.	Acknowledge that they are both there today. Be alert for why this might be. Ask about thoughts/ fears/hopes. Involve them both in the consultation.	Missing the main point of the consultation so the patient and/or partner leaves dissatisfied.
The patient looks uncomfortable and tense as they walk through the door.	There is something that they are worried about or find difficulty in saying. If this hasn't yet come across in the consultation, ask:	'I noticed that you looked a little bit tense when you came in the room tonight and I just wondered if there was anything else that might be troubling you?'	You miss the point of the consultation and either they tell you the difficulty late in the consultation or they come back for another one soon afterwards.
The patient says, 'The first thing I want to tell you about is ...'.	There is something else! There may even be more than two problems. It is very easy to miss the fact that the patient said, 'The first thing ...' as you can get absorbed in the details of the problem they are describing.	At a suitable moment early in the consultation but when they seem to have come to a natural pause, ask 'You said that was the first thing ... can I just ask you if there was something else that you would like us to deal with today?'	You spend 10 minutes dealing with the first problem. Only then do they mention the second one.
The patient who consults very rarely but has come three times in the last month with minor symptoms of trivial illness.	Again, there is something worrying the patient that they haven't yet been able to tell you.	You could reflect the behaviour: 'You know, you're someone who doesn't come to see us very often, but I'm aware that you've come in three times in the last month and I'm just wondering if there was anything else troubling you that you haven't yet mentioned?'	They will continue to consult with minor matters until someone picks up the cue that there may be more to this than meets the eye.

Table 7.1 (Continued)

Cue	What it might mean	Examples of what you might say or do	Pitfalls of missing the cue
The teenager who comes (possibly with a friend) and asks for help with heavy periods.	A classic presentation of a teenager who would like to go on the Pill but isn't able to ask directly for it. She may well already be sexually active and worried about pregnancy.	Needs sensitive handling and awareness of all the possibilities: 'One way of managing heavy periods is to take the contraceptive Pill. I was wondering if that's something that you had been thinking about?'	She goes away with her needs unmet and at risk of an unplanned pregnancy.
When a patient repeats a word or phrase more than once, for example: 'worried', 'stress'.	They are concerned that they may have a stress-related problem or anxiety or another mental health problem, but don't know quite how to express this.	'You've mentioned the word "stress" twice and I was wondering whether you feel you are under stress at the moment?'	You may miss the patient's main concerns.
The patient whose eyes mist up briefly when in the middle of telling you something and they move swiftly on to a different area.	Quite clearly something is upsetting them, but they are either unwilling or unable to talk freely about it.	'I noticed that you seemed a little upset when you were telling me about ...' (said in a caring way, and tentatively in case the patient really doesn't want to talk about it).	You lose the opportunity to deepen your understanding of the patient and their problems.

Cues generally need to be checked out with the patient – after all, the patient who scratches their head may simply have an itchy scalp! You can acknowledge cues as soon as you notice them. This has immediacy and ensures that they are not missed, but you may well break the patient's train of thought or take them down blind alleys (or interesting, but irrelevant byways). You can hold onto them until a suitable moment, but you run the risk of forgetting them altogether. It takes practice and skill to listen to the patient's unfolding story, note the cues, but hang onto them and then refer to them in a helpful way.

Cues may take several forms:

Non-verbal
- how the patient looks when they come in the room (clothes, gait, eye contact)
- how the patient sits down (slowly, eyes cast down, confidently, in visible pain)
- the messages from the patient's musculoskeletal system as they are telling their story (squirming, sitting very still, wringing their hands).

Verbal

- how the patient delivers their words (tone of voice, pitch, rate of speech)
- repetition of key words or phrases
- use of emotionally-laden words such as 'worried', 'stress', 'not coping', 'depressed'.

Verbal and non-verbal

- a mismatch between words and musculoskeletal system (sad words delivered with a smile, words that depict extreme anxiety or stress delivered with serenity).

Other

- two parents bringing a child
- the patient who rarely attends, but has been several times in the last few weeks
- the patient who brings a partner or friend with them.

Use of silence

Silence can be a surprisingly powerful listening tool. If there is an awkward pause in the consultation, it can be tempting to fill it with a useful question or statement. A good use of time in a busy morning's surgery? Perhaps, but letting the patient fill the silence instead is even more useful. Clinicians who are fairly new to the job sometimes find silences unbearable and interminably long, and become overwhelmed with the need to say something. Biting your tongue and holding back will almost always mean that the patient will speak into the silence instead, potentially a real eye-opener that gives both clinician and patient new insights.

The silence usually feels much longer than it is and, if you video or audiotape your surgeries, you can time the length of any silence. However long it felt at the time, it is rare for it to last more than 20 seconds – and the rewards may be considerable!

Softening

When you are trying to find out information from patients (remembering that this may be difficult, embarrassing or anxiety-provoking for them, even if you have heard it all before), it can be worth having a repertoire of ways that you can soften questions or statements. Softeners are phrases that you can use at the beginning of a sentence in order to take the edge off any sense of interrogation, for example:

- 'You know, I was just wondering whether ...'
- 'Would you mind if I asked you ...'
- 'Is it OK if I ask you some more about this?'
- 'Thinking about it now ...'

Taking the edge off a question by using a softener can help to get underneath a patient's natural defence mechanisms (the internal policemen) and find out where the real difficulty lies. It's much easier to help them when you know what's really troubling them. For example, you might be wondering whether a middle-aged businessman with dysuria has actually contracted a sexually transmitted infection. The real question sounds harsh or aggressive and might well be confrontational:

- 'Do you think you have picked up a sexually transmitted infection?'
- 'Have you had sex with a prostitute?'
- 'Have you been unfaithful to your partner?'

These questions might provoke a knee-jerk, 'No – certainly not!' even if the real answer is 'Yes'. Instead you might use a softener to take the edge off the harshness: 'I know you go to the Far East a lot ... I was just wondering whether you had been tempted to have a sexual relationship with someone there.'

This is now a statement rather than a question, so it doesn't have to be answered at all. Paradoxically, this makes it easier for the patient to answer because it takes the pressure off. 'I was just wondering' is the softener and implies a tentative thought that you are merely checking out with the patient and you would be quite happy to be told that you are wrong. The main verb in the above sentence is now 'tempted' rather than 'have sex'. The patient might be willing to say 'yes' to 'tempted' and from there reveal that the temptation led to action. In other words they can tell you a little bit of the story first and see how you respond to it and, if you don't appear too shocked or horrified, they might well be able to tell you the rest.

Lewis Walker (2002) describes the use of softeners in much more detail and gives lots of very useful examples to try.

My friend John/Jane

This technique was first described by Milton Erickson, an American therapist (Haley, 1973). It involves describing the problem as if it belonged to someone else, in other words placing a verbal safety barrier between the patient and a potentially difficult question. You need to second-guess or have a hunch about what it might be that's really troubling the patient and that they're finding it hard to tell you about. For example:

- 'You know, someone I know – a good friend – went through a really rough time too when ...'
- 'I've sometimes found that patients who have the sort of symptoms that you've been telling me about are secretly worried that they've got AIDS/a sexually transmitted disease/something really horrible/cancer, even. I'm just wondering whether that might possibly be something that you, too, are worrying about?'
- 'You know, many people in your shoes might feel very upset/pretty angry/really quite worried and I'm just wondering if that's how you are feeling as well?'

Sleeping policemen

This is nothing to do with those bumps in the road designed to make you slow down! All of us have internal 'policemen' that help us, generally, to conform to what society expects, and not to break social rules too often. These policemen stop us (most of us, most of the time at least) from:

- telling Mr Smith that he is a boring overweight moaner and that you are completely fed up with him coming to see you
- visibly ogling a stranger in the street and telling them that they are incredibly attractive

- standing up in the theatre and shouting 'rubbish' (even if it is)
- stripping off in the middle of the street because it's hot.

Clearly, the internal policemen help us to behave in a generally conforming way in society and stop the external policemen from arresting us for unprofessional, bizarre, antisocial or threatening behaviour!

Sometimes the internal policemen prevent patients from telling us that they are really worried about something because they are scared of the consequences. But sometimes, in consultations, the internal policemen can be off guard or briefly fall asleep long enough for the patient's fears to slip out underneath. Watching consultation videos can be a very good way of spotting this. Times when the patient's internal policemen seem to be particularly off guard are the 'in-between' times. In other words, the fears tend to be well under control when you and the patient are in dialogue together but slip out like ghosts in the night through the cracks and spaces between the phases of the consultation. These include:

- the moment that the patient stands up to walk over to the examination couch
- when you have your stethoscope in your ears and are checking their blood pressure or listening to their heart or chest, etc
- when you are touching them but they can't see you directly, for example when you are listening to the back of their chest
- when you are looking at the computer screen to read their past notes or to check what drugs they are taking
- when you are turned away from them, washing your hands, getting the auriscope, etc
- when they are dressing after you have examined them, particularly if you and they are on opposite sides of the screen
- when you are busy writing a prescription, sick note or request form or entering information on the computer.

Of course, these are the times that you are also likely to be a bit off guard too and not really giving the patient 100% of your attention. Some phrases that I have heard slip out in these moments (and that are only too easy to overlook whilst you are thinking about what is going on, working out what to do or say next, or generally engaged with other tasks) are:

- 'I hope it's nothing serious.'
- 'My mother had cancer.'
- 'I hope it's not my heart.'
- 'My neighbour dropped dead.'
- 'I've been thinking I should come.'
- 'People don't get TB any more, do they?'
- 'My husband's been at me for ages to come.'
- 'I might lose my job.'
- 'I've been so worried.'

Sometimes these are disguised with a small laugh or even a joke, for example: 'I've not been myself at all since she was born' (ha-ha)(a new mother, bringing her 4-month-old baby with a minor viral illness).

It's worth having your consultation antennae tuned in so that you can hear these anxieties that slip past the internal policemen, and can give them the proper attention they deserve. This is not the moment to ignore them (consciously or unconsciously) or idly laugh along with the patient at their not-at-all-funny joke.

Noticing when the internal policemen are on duty

The in-between bits of the consultation are times when the internal policemen can briefly be off guard and fall asleep. There are other points in the consultation when you can get a sense that the internal policemen are very much awake and active, and are actively restraining something that the patient in front of you might possibly want to say.

Signs that the policemen are active and therefore that there may well be something worrying the patient that they are having difficulty telling you are when the patient:

- who has been talking fluently and freely, starts to hesitate with pauses, gaps or mumbling
- may giggle, tremble or become tearful
- becomes flushed, squirms, shuffles or adjusts their position
- falls completely silent and seems to have 'gone inside'.

Bypassing the internal policemen

Of course, the first thing is to notice when patients hesitate and to start raising your alertness whenever this happens. What you do next will determine whether you find out more or lose the opportunity.

Helpful behaviour

- Stay in rapport with the patient.
- Look interested, leaning forward, nodding, etc.
- Ask gentle questions or give prompts:
  - 'Tell me a bit more.'
  - 'I can see/hear/feel this is difficult for you.'
  - 'I'm interested to hear more about that.'
- Gently repeat the exact word or few words that the patient has just used.

Unhelpful behaviour

- Breaking rapport by turning away, for example to the computer or to get out a sick note or stethoscope.
- Changing the subject, perhaps because you are uncomfortable with what's going on. Remember this may well be the patient's discomfort that has got displaced to you in a counter-transference process.
- Firing questions that you would like to know the answers to (and may well need to ask at some stage), but that aren't directly related to what the patient is saying at this moment, for example 'How is your appetite? What's your sleep pattern? What medication do you take? How is your wife?'

What to do when you notice that the patient has 'gone inside'

You will recognise this when some or all of the following signs are present:

- the patient's speech has become less and less fluent until it has stopped, possibly in the middle of a sentence
- instead of looking at you or looking round the room, they are looking down
- their breathing may be slightly different, shallower and slightly more rapid.

This means that the patient's attention is entirely focused on themselves and their internal world. What is happening? They may well be (internally) visiting places in their past or other things in their lives and may be making new connections.

What should you do? As little as possible! Sit still, pay attention, look at the patient, perhaps alter your own breathing slightly so that it matches the rise and fall of the patient's. Above all, it is really important to stay in non-verbal rapport and not interrupt their search process. Sometimes clinicians interrupt, often because they are uncomfortable and desperate to replace silence with words. They may ask a question. Doing this will drag the patient out of their internal world and right back into the room. They will almost certainly lose their thread and the moment for important connections will have been lost.

Instead, sit with the patient and wait until they come back into the present. You will recognise this because they will look up, their eyes will start to focus again and they may make a physical gesture such as a sigh or brief shake of the head. Now is the moment to pay complete attention to the patient, to have your antennae tuned in and use all your best listening skills. If you do this and look interested, they will almost certainly tell you spontaneously what they have been thinking about and where they have just been.

> 'You know ... it's really odd. I've just been thinking about when I was a kid and I would sit on the stairs whilst my dad hit my mum and she cried – I got headaches then too – haven't thought about that for years.'

If they don't, you could ask 'What were you thinking about just now?'

It is worth paying very close attention to what the patient says when they emerge from this internal search. As Roger Neighbour (1987) says, it's an opportunity to find gold nuggets near the surface.

Ideas, concerns and expectations

These three are the 'holy trinity' of patient-centred consultations. Finding out information from people is more than finding out what has happened to them already to bring them in to see you (i.e. past information). It's also about working out where they are in the here-and-now and what their thoughts are about the future.

Ideas

Just as each clinician has their own consultation model, every patient will have their own illness and health model. This will be informed from all sorts of different sources, some of them more reliable than others! For example:

- past experience
- experiences of friends or relatives
- articles in the newspaper or the women's magazine at the hairdressers
- the Internet
- factual programmes on the television
- fictional programmes on the television, such as Holby City, ER, Casualty, Bodies.

So it is well worth asking the question (and phrasing it in whatever way works for you):

- 'What thoughts have you already had about this?'
- 'You've had these symptoms for a few weeks now, so what's been going through your mind?'

Whatever they say, and however implausible or unlikely, listen, nod and stay in rapport rather than challenging at this stage. You could summarise back to them so that they and you are quite clear about their understanding. Hold on to what they say so that you can return to it when explaining and planning.

Concerns

'What are you worrying about, then?'

If you ask it like that, most patients will say 'nothing' which isn't true or they will pussyfoot around something that is not very worrying at all and which you rightly suspect is not the real problem. Some more useful questions are:

- 'You seem concerned about this' (a statement being used as a question)
- 'Is there anything (however unlikely) that you are particularly worried this might be?'
- 'Sometimes, in the middle of the night, all of us have worries about symptoms. Is there anything that you have been worrying about in the dark?'

It can also be helpful to use 'My friend John' in reverse:

- 'I'm wondering what your partner/husband/wife thinks about this.'
- 'When you've talked with your friends about this, are there any particular worries that they have expressed?'

You can only reassure patients if you know what they are worrying about. I cannot emphasise this too strongly! If you reassure them about what you think or guess they are worrying about, you will get it wrong and be ineffective most of the time.

Example 1

Mum brings Kylie, aged 6, who has a persistent and bad cough at night. The clinician makes an assumption that the problem is a chest infection or possibly asthma and launches into their stock speech: 'This is a viral illness, which will get better on its own ...', followed by an explanation and reassurance that it isn't asthma. The mother was actually worried about whether it was whooping cough as Kylie had reacted badly to her first triple immunisation and not had the rest of the course. This only became clear the following week when she brought her daughter back.

Example 2

Lucy, a 19-year-old single mum brings Tyler, her one-year-old baby, to see you in evening surgery. She had consulted the nurse practitioner this morning and the notes read: 'Diarrhoea for 1 day. No vomiting. Well baby.

Temp normal. Not dehydrated. Advised clear fluids for 24 hours and to stay off milk.'

The symptoms are no different but Lucy seems worried. As you start to unpick the worry, you notice that she looks very anxious and that she says twice, 'I'm worried he won't take his milk.' Asking her the question, 'And if he doesn't take his milk ...?' leads to the following series of responses.

> **Patient:** Well, all babies need their milk, don't they?
> **Doctor:** They need their milk because ...?
> **Patient:** Otherwise they won't get the food they need ...
> **Doctor:** And if they don't get the food they need ...?
> **Patient:** Their brains won't grow properly.
> **Doctor:** And if their brain doesn't grow properly ... ?
> **Patient:** Then he'll get brain damage (bursts into tears).
> **Doctor:** Can I just check I've got this right? (clarifying and checking). You're worried that giving him just water and juice and cutting right down on the milk might mean that he ends up with brain damage?
> **Patient:** Yes! (loud, clear and positive; everything about her communication, verbal and non-verbal, was stating 'Yes!')

So Tyler's mum was worried that he would get brain damage from the diarrhoea. This is such a remote possibility that few reasonable health professionals would give it a second thought and would certainly not offer reassurance about this routinely. Having got this (very real) worry out into the open, it was then relatively quick and easy to refute it and defuse the situation – and Tyler and his mum left much more confident about what they were doing.

Expectations

This is about the future. What do patients think or hope that you are going to do? Finding out can save you a lot of wasted effort!

Example – a cautionary tale

I recently watched a consultation video in which an articulate elderly lady described knee pain. The doctor used a competent and skilful set of open and closed questions and did a thorough physical examination to find out about the problem. He then launched into an articulate, comprehensive and detailed verbal description of a hierarchy of treatment for osteoarthritis of the knee:

> '... simple analgesics like aspirin or paracetamol, physiotherapy, non-steroidal anti-inflammatory drugs like ibuprofen (though, of course, we would need to be careful because of your age and the fact that your kidneys aren't so good), Cox 2 inhibitors (used to

be the best thing since sliced bread but they've had some bad publicity recently), knee replacement surgery (though this would be a last resort, of course)'.

The patient listened patiently nodding politely and all this went on for several minutes. Eventually the doctor came to the crux of this speech, gave a broad smile, asked (with the MRCGP exam firmly in his mind), 'What would you like to do?' and paused expectantly. The patient looked him straight back in the eye and said: 'But I only wanted to know what it was; it really isn't bad enough to need any treatment at all'.

If the doctor had found this out in the first place, a lot of time and effort could have been saved!

So it is well worth formulating a question along the lines of:

- 'Tell me, what did you have in mind that I might be able to do for you today?'
- 'When you booked the appointment/were on the way to see me today/were sitting in the waiting room, was there anything in particular that you hoped that I might be able to do for you?'

You will notice that each of these is preceded by a degree of 'softening'. The real question, here, is of course: 'What do you want me to do?' And, if you challenge your patients with that bald and unsoftened question, you can hardly be surprised if you get a rather tart and swift reply: 'That's what I came to find out!' or 'You're the doctor/nurse – you tell me!' As usual, the key to asking this question in a helpful way and getting useful information from the patient is rapport.

When you are stuck

There are some consultations when you are reasonably sure that there is more going on than you have found out so far. Perhaps there is incongruity between the patient's words and their non-verbal behaviour. Or it may be that the parrot on your shoulder is whispering to you: 'You're missing something!' Some useful questions that you could try include:

- 'When was the last time you felt this way?' (using the patient's feelings to make connections with past events)
- 'Who else in the family is worried about your symptoms?' (helping to place the problem within the context of the family and is also an oblique use of 'my friend John')
- 'I have a feeling that I may be missing something, but I'm not quite sure what it is' (making your own feelings explicit may help the patient to do the same).

Possible action points

- Make a list of the skills described in this chapter. Think about your consultations (even better, video some of them and watch them either alone or with someone who is willing to help you reflect). Map which skills you use by ticking them off each time you use them. If you find there are some skills that you use very rarely, or not at all, make a conscious effort to incorporate these into each consultation in a surgery.

- As you become fluent in an underused skill and it starts to move into the arena of 'unconscious competence', think about adding in another new skill.
- Try finding out from every patient in a morning's surgery what they are really worried about. Everyone I know who has tried this has been surprised at some very unexpected responses.
- Be on the look out for the policemen, sleeping or awake, and practise being especially alert to what the patient is saying or not saying at these times.
- Watch for the 'cracks in the consultation'. What emerges from them?

References and further reading

- Haley J. *Uncommon Therapy: psychiatric techniques of Milton II Erickson MD*. New York: WW Norton and Co Ltd; 1973, reprinted 1993.
- Neighbour R. *The Inner Consultation*. Lancaster: MTP Press; 1987. 2nd edn Oxford: Radcliffe Publishing; 2004.
- Walker L. *Consulting with NLP*. Oxford: Radcliffe Medical Press; 2002.

Chapter 8

Summarising and reflecting

Proust's novel ostensibly tells of the irrevocability of time lost, the forfeiture of innocence through experience, the reinstatement of extra-temporal values of time regained, ultimately the novel is both optimistic and set within the context of a humane religious experience, re-stating as it does the concept of intemporality.

'Monty Python's Flying Circus – Summarize Proust' (in 15 seconds) competition (BBC first shown 16 November 1972)

Key points

- It is easy to miss out this stage of the consultation but using it will pay dividends.
- Summarising will generally shorten, rather than lengthen, a consultation by avoiding blind alleys and false trails.
- It helps patients to realise that you have heard what they said and to add any missing pieces of information before you move together towards a management plan.
- In this way, summarising is like a fulcrum or pivotal point in the consultation.

This is part of the consultation that can easily get forgotten. It's all too easy to decide that you've worked out what's wrong with the patient and move into a management plan, leaving out this 'unnecessary' and 'time consuming' stage of summarising. But there are two very good reasons for summarising:

- summarising is a very efficient way of using time and can shorten the consultation, whilst improving its quality
- many consultations that might go wrong can be retrieved if the clinician reflects and summarises back to the patient before moving on.

Example

OK – so can I just check that I've got this right? You've been feeling increasingly tired and have had no energy for months, you've lost a bit of weight and had this funny pain in your back. You've been worrying about it for quite a few weeks, not sure whether to come and see us or not, but the last straw was when your daughter came round and said you looked awful and insisted that you do something.

It's particularly important to use the patient's language – nouns, verbs and representational states – when doing this. Being the patient, on the receiving end of someone's summary, is a very positive experience.

- It shows you that the doctor or nurse has been listening to you.
- The way that they say the words (hopefully, at least!) demonstrates that they are caring and interested, and aren't belittling your symptoms or fears.
- It helps you to realise that they have got hold of everything that you said so that you can have some degree of confidence that they are able to take all your symptoms or problems into account.
- You can even gain new insights into any difficulties or problems by hearing them stated by someone else. It is particularly worth noting that this is much easier if the summariser uses your words rather than theirs.

When you summarise, it may be a straightforward précis of what the patient said without much in the way of interpretation. But sometimes you can add tentative interpretations – perhaps you know the patient and can make connections for her that she hasn't seen for herself, or you may be able to connect two or more parts of the story in a helpful and interpretative way.

Example

Mrs C has told the clinician about a number of recent life events that have left her feeling weepy and tired. The clinician summarises back:

> You've told me about being made redundant, then your mother died and there was a burglary at home the same week. The last straw was when the dog died ... (straightforward summary)
> ... You've had a lot of sad things happen recently. (interpretation), OR
> ... and I'm remembering that your dad died last year and you became quite low after that. (linking present symptoms to past knowledge of the patient)

When you summarise, it's very important to watch and listen to the patient attentively all the time; just as important as when she told you the story in the first place. As you speak, your words may fall on fertile ground and the patient will nod and agree. At other times it may be clear that you have missed the point or made a near miss. Many patients will interject as you are going along and add their own contributions, help to clarify details or make minor corrections if you've got it wrong. So summarising is not a passive, mechanical delivery of words from one person to another, but often a very dynamic process in which both clinician and patient construct a shared overview of the problem.

When you have finished your summary, leave a space, remain very attentive and watch the patient's response to this. She may say 'yes' in a way that is very clear and positive, so that you know you can move on to the next part of the consultation. In the jargon, there is a set of behaviours that is called a 'yes set', in which everything about the patient's communication, verbal and non-verbal, is saying that she positively agrees with you. When you get to this point, you have got there! You and the patient understand each other.

If you haven't got a very clear, unmistakeable 'yes', you've got a 'no'. This doesn't have to be the actual word 'no' – it is frequently some variant that may even, superficially, sound like 'yes'. The variants include: 'yes ...', 'er ... yes ...', 'yes, but ...', 'er ... sort of ...'. Clearly you are on the right lines but you haven't got there yet! A partial yes is a 'no' and tells you that the patient needs to say more. She can now do so.

- 'I think I ought to tell you something else. Erm ... it's a bit embarrassing ... but I've been, you know, passing blood as well.'
- 'Erm ... I'm not sure how to tell you this but ... I had sex with someone else.'
- 'I've been so worried it's cancer.'

One reason that patients feel dissatisfied or only partially satisfied with consultations, and/or return for another one within a short space of time is that they haven't told the clinician everything that was worrying them. They may not even have realised this at the time; sometimes the anxiety only surfaces when they have had a chance to think and reflect, perhaps when they are back home talking with their partner. Summarising enables patients to reflect for themselves during the consultation, whilst they still have chance to express their worries.

Sometimes it also gives you the opportunity to put the consultation back on track. You may not have made a near miss so much as got it completely wrong. It is so much easier if you find this out part way through the consultation rather than right at the end or, much worse, when the letter of complaint arrives!

Possible action points

- If you are not in the habit of using summaries, start practising them. It's worth starting with relatively straightforward consultations and then moving on to ones where you have been given a lot of information to hold onto.
- Start watching for a 'yes set', not just in consultations but also in social conversations and interactions with people.
- Once you can clearly recognise a 'yes set', start looking out for a 'not quite yes set' and see if you can work out what's missing.

References and further reading

- Neighbour R. *The Inner Consultation*. Lancaster: MTP Press; 1987. 2nd edn Oxford: Radcliffe Publishing; 2004.
- Walker L. *Consulting with NLP*. Oxford: Radcliffe Medical Press; 2002.

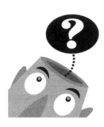

Chapter 9

Giving information to patients

The hours of non-hours work worked by a worker in a pay reference period shall be the total of the number of hours spent by him during the pay reference period in carrying out the duties required of him under his contract to do non-hours work.

(Draft National Minimum Wage Regulations 1998, voted the worst example of gobbledygook by worldwide supporters of the Plain English Campaign)

I know you believe you understood what I think I said but I am not sure you realise that what you heard is not what I meant.

(Author unknown, variously attributed)

Key points

- In most consultations you need to give information of some sort to patients.
- Patients will be able to hear and take in information most effectively when:
  - it is delivered in small pieces
  - you check understanding before moving on
  - you use language that matches theirs (nouns and representational states)
  - you deliver it at the right speed or pace.
- The right side of the brain can only hear the nouns, verbs and descriptive words that you use. It can't hear the word 'not'.

At some stage of most consultations it is likely that you will need to give information to patients. There are a number of different variations on this theme, including:

- telling them what you think is wrong with them (including, of course, breaking bad news)
- explaining what a letter from the hospital means
- interpreting blood or other test results
- telling them that they need a referral or to go to the hospital for tests
- describing the treatment plan to them
- explaining how to take medication.

These different sorts of information-giving require a portfolio of skills. There are some skills that are common to all of them:

- maintaining rapport
- using language well
- delivering the information in manageable pieces
- checking that patients have understood what you've said
- pacing your delivery.

Maintaining rapport

Generally, information is given in the second part of the consultation. If you have worked at building and maintaining rapport throughout the consultation, you should be well and truly on the same wavelength as the patient by the time you get to this point. Mutual rapport will also make it easier for the patient to take in and assimilate what you are saying.

Using language well

This is the first time in the consultation when it is likely that you will do more talking than the patient. If you have paid attention to the patient's representational system and health vocabulary, you should now have a good idea about which nouns and verbs to use.

Another skill is to phrase information positively and avoid using negatives such as 'no', 'not' and 'don't'. There are several reasons for this:

* communication is clearer if you say 'do' rather than 'don't'. 'Take these tablets' is as clear as it can be. 'Don't forget to take the tablets' is less clear as it introduces two different things to do – 'take the tablets' and 'forget to take the tablets'
* saying 'no', 'not' and 'don't' immediately opens up possibilities for behaviour that may not have occurred to the patient.

Well-meaning clinicians sometimes fall into the trap of using negative words and phrases and, paradoxically, this can have the opposite effect from that intended. 'This won't hurt!' is meant well and often precedes some sort of examination that is very familiar to the clinician (for example, examination of the abdomen or looking in a child's ear) but not, perhaps, to the patient. If the patient hadn't thought, even for a moment, that it might be painful, they will now recognise that it might be and may tense up. Instead you could use better alternatives:

* 'You'll just feel my hand touching you.'
* 'This may feel tickly.'

'You mustn't stop the antidepressants until I see you again in two weeks time' is also unhelpful. Even though the patient might nod and agree that they won't stop them, you have introduced the possibility that they might do so. A different way of putting it might be:

* 'The antidepressants take a while to work. It's important to take them each day for the next two weeks, even though you may feel no different at first. When I see you in a fortnight you can tell me how you've been getting on.'

'I know you're self-employed, but you really can't go to work next week' almost invites a free spirit to be defiant! 'Says who, mate? Don't you tell me what to do! What do you know about being self-employed anyway?'

You could try an alternative, more empathic approach, which is also more likely to get results:

* 'Like you, I'm self-employed and I know it can be hard to take time off to rest. But if you look after yourself next week, you will get better more quickly.'

Let me give you another example:

> 'For the next minute, I want you to make sure that you don't think about giraffes. Please don't conjure up a picture in your head of a tall giraffe, in the plains of Africa, reaching its long neck to pull leaves from a tree. Definitely no giraffes. After all, there aren't any giraffes around here at all, are there? Please clear your mind of all giraffes. OK?'

I bet you weren't thinking about giraffes five minutes ago!

In the above examples, what the brain hears are messages like these:

- 'This will hurt.'
- 'Stop the antidepressants.'
- 'Go to work next week.'
- 'Think about giraffes.'

These are powerful subliminal messages and may mean that the outcome is exactly opposite to the one you intended. Try, instead using only positive words with no 'don'ts, mustn'ts, or can'ts' in them.

- 'You'll just feel me touching you.'
- 'Remember to take the tablets each day.'
- 'Stay off work and rest for the next 10 days.'
- 'Think about how what you are reading relates to your consultations.'

Delivering the information in manageable pieces – 'chunks'

If someone gave you a very large chocolate bar, assuming you like chocolate, you might be eager to eat it. How would you do this? It's likely that you'd want to break a few pieces off first and just make sure that it is to your taste before you polish off the whole lot. Anyway, it would be difficult to stuff the bar into your mouth all at once. In the same way, most advice needs breaking down into bite-sized chunks in order to make it digestible. As you deliver each chunk of information to the patient, watch them to see how it's going down. Are they hungry for more or overwhelmed? Do you need to make the chunks smaller or larger?

Checking that patients have understood what you've said – '... and check'

Most health professionals think that they explain things in a way that patients can understand. They then hope that patients have understood what they've said and, if you asked them, might well tell you that they definitely do check patients' understanding. Watching consultation videos is revealing; the majority of doctors and nurses either don't check understanding, relying on the fact that the patient is sitting there, nodding and not actually disagreeing, or they use a phrase that they believe checks understanding, but doesn't, such as: 'Is that OK?', 'Is that clear?', 'Got it?' And – guess what – patients almost invariably nod and say 'Yes!'

It's really hard for patients to answer 'no' or ask for more clarification when faced with a health professional who is asking a question that is begging for a knee-jerk 'yes'. If you actually bother to check what they have understood, there may well be whole chunks that they miss out altogether and other bits that are just plain wrong.

Sometimes clinicians worry about sounding condescending or patronising and struggle to find a form of words that effectively asks the patient to repeat back to them what they have just said. Here are some useful approaches.

- 'I know I've given you a lot of information in a short space of time – just run through what I've said to you so that I know you've got it.'
- 'Now I know that I don't always explain things as well/as clearly as I'd like to, so would you mind just telling me what you've understood that I've said, so that I'll know if there's any bits we should go through again.'
- 'OK – do you mind if I ask you to just go over that for me, so that I know that I've been clear enough and that you've got hold of what I was trying to say?'
- 'Just so that I'm clear that you know what you are doing, tell me what you might say about this to your wife/husband when you go home tonight.'

It's well worth working out a form of words that works for you and that conveys the following message.

- It's quite OK if you haven't yet heard or understood everything I've said.
- If you haven't, it's not in any way because you are stupid, inattentive or a bad listener.
- It's probably because I haven't explained things clearly enough or just that there was a lot of information.
- I'm happy to tell you again and I'd much rather do this than have you go away confused or having only partially understood.

And once again, as with so many other parts of the consultation, the key to being able to say this effectively so that the patient feels that the clinician cares that they understand rather than feels patronised or belittled is rapport.

It's worth working out some phrases that are authentic for you, and that sound and feel right and work for you. If you don't normally check understanding, have a go. The results might be surprising and you may discover that this is something that you need to start using more often.

Pacing

Pacing means getting the delivery of your information at the right speed for the patient. On the one hand you probably want to use time as effectively as possible, but on the other hand if you rush, the patient will not take in much of what you say so that the time you do spend with them will be less effective. So, how can you judge pace?

Patients teach you the pace that they can handle – if you only listen for it! Think back to the early part of the consultation when the patient was giving *you* information. At the time, you may have been concentrating on the content rather than the delivery, but if you also paid attention to their delivery and pace, then you would have been able to deduce how quickly or slowly the patient manages information.

If you speak any faster than they do or try to give them information at a faster rate, they will miss bits of what you say because they won't be able to take it in at that speed. You may need to slow your speech for some patients or deliver chunks of information fairly slowly.

As you give information, make sure you are watching and listening all the time for the patient's minimal cues. What are the clues telling you?

- Is the patient engaged with you and processing information?
- Or do they seem doubtful or hesitant?
- Have they got 'stuck' trying to make sense of something that wasn't at all clear to them so that they are now thinking about this and unable to take in anything else that you are saying?
- Are you going too fast so they are missing bits ...?
- Or too slow so that they are bored and you are both wasting time?
- Do you need to stop and check anything with them?

If it's apparent that the patient is not fully engaged with you, you must stop and check it out with them.

- 'You're looking a bit puzzled.'
- 'I'm wondering if I'm going too fast.'
- 'How does that sound to you?'
- 'Let me just check that you're clear so far.'

Specific skills for giving different types of information

Telling people what you think is wrong with them

When telling people what you think is wrong, it is really helpful to know what they have already thought themselves and what their fears are. So their responses to questions that you have already asked when finding out information will be a good starting point. For example, you may have asked:

- 'And, tell me, have you had any thoughts about this yourself?'
- 'Is there anything that, however unlikely, you are worrying might be wrong with you?'

Patients' responses to these questions give you an easy place to start. This is the point in the consultation when you can really make use of this information that you have learnt from them and have been holding onto until this point:

- 'You told me that you wondered whether you might have a chest infection and I think you may well be right.'
- 'You mentioned that you thought you might be developing tonsillitis and need antibiotics. I think, myself, that it's actually much more likely that your sore throat is being caused by a virus. It doesn't look like tonsillitis and I don't think that antibiotics would help – in fact they might make you feel worse.'
- 'Now I know you mentioned that you were worried that this was skin cancer and I'm pleased to say that I'm pretty sure it isn't.'

Remember to use the patient's own nouns, verbs and representational system, so you can match their health dialect.

Thinking aloud

Another useful skill is to think aloud. Let the patient share in your thought process. You might start by summarising back the symptoms and the findings, and then let them follow your train of thought so they know how you've come to the point you eventually arrive at. This can make the diagnosis seem much clearer and lets the patient feel that they have been a part of the process of getting there. It also empowers patients and stops you being perceived as a magician who conjures up clever diagnoses out of a top hat. Patients may also feel more able to challenge what you've said or tell you about their fears about what's wrong if you are open and clear with them.

> 'You've had a really bad, stabbing pain in the top part of your stomach (patient's own words) that was worse after drinking alcohol and you wondered if it might be an ulcer or even stomach cancer. Now you're only 25 so that would be really very young to get stomach cancer and you haven't lost weight or anything like that. An ulcer is possible, but again it would be rare in someone of your age. It's much more likely that the alcohol irritated your stomach and has given you some inflammation – called gastritis.'

Explaining what a letter from the hospital means

Some consultations start with 'I wondered if you've heard from Dr X at the hospital yet?'. With luck, you have heard and the letter is filed electronically or in the paper record in front of you. How are you going to tell the patient what it says? A good place to start is to acknowledge that you have got the letter and are happy to discuss it and add, 'but tell me first what happened when you went to the clinic and what Dr X said to you'. This is useful because it is likely to give you clues both about what happened in the hospital consultation (particularly if it was at all rushed or dysfunctional), but also about what the patient has understood (or misunderstood). It may also tell why they've come today and help to shape the rest of the consultation. You will notice if they are anxious or distressed, so that you can tailor your response appropriately.

Do you let patients read or have copies of hospital letters written about them? Some consultants copy patients into their letters and others write their primary letter to the patient, with a copy for information to the GP. Others don't and the GP is the only person to get a copy of the letter. Patients are, of course, entitled to see their own medical records and, if you have the computer screen turned towards the patient, it is quite likely that they will read some or all of the letter anyway. If they can partially see the letter, it may be helpful to print off a copy and give it to them, or at least to go through the letter on the computer screen with them. If you decide to do this, read the letter aloud with the patient and check that they understand both the words and the meaning, and also that what is written is an accurate representation of what happened!

Interpreting blood or other test results for patients

Imagine you have been worried enough about your health to visit your GP and they have sent you to the hospital for a blood test, ultrasound, chest X-ray or something similar. You are now even more worried about what might be wrong. After all, the doctor or nurse clearly didn't know what was wrong from listening to your symptoms and examining you, and needed to find out more. This means (to you) that there is at least a chance that it is something more serious than you had feared. You go back for the results either by prior arrangement or because a receptionist has phoned you and told you to come in; by now you are really very worried.

There are two features of this sort of consultation that set it apart from others.

- You should probably avoid a minimalist type of opening. If you just smile and nod at the patient and invite them to sit down, there may well follow an uncomfortable and difficult silence in which you think the patient is going to open the consultation and the patient believes that you will. So you might need to launch straight in with a greeting like 'Hello there – nice to see you again', followed by a brief pause. This gives the opportunity for the patient to say anything pressing or urgent. If the patient just looks expectantly, then you can carry on with checking out that they have come today for their results.
- The second problem is that it may be difficult to build rapport early. If it starts either with the patient saying, 'I've come for my test results' or 'The receptionist said to make an appointment' or you saying, 'Now then – I think you're here for your results?', then the usual opportunity to build rapport whilst letting the patient do most of the talking is lost. You will also be in the difficult situation of giving information without having checked the patient's understanding about the situation or their hopes and fears.

Many patients coming for test results are anxious and some will be worried sick. If the test is normal, it is as well to say this straight away: 'I'm very pleased to be able to tell you that everything is fine/normal/OK.'

You may then want to go into the detail, but much better to do it this way round than have the patient worrying whilst you read the report aloud to them.

> 'Yes ... well, your haemoglobin is normal ... and your white cells? Let me see ... er ... yes ... they are OK too. Er, let me look at your kidney function ... just a minute whilst I find the right page ... well, er ... these seem fine too ...'

It is excruciating to be on the receiving end of this!

If there is something that needs attention but is not too significant, you can give an overview first.

> 'Pretty much everything is fine, but we have found out why you've been so tired lately and I'm pleased to say it's something we should be able to sort out relatively easily.'

If there is a real problem, then you may need some 'breaking bad news' skills.

Explaining how to take medication

Some of the generic skills of giving information are essential here:

- phrasing it positively: 'Remember to take the tablets until I see you next'
- checking understanding: 'Just tell me how you're going to take the tablets, so that I know I've explained it well enough'.

Describing the treatment plan to patients

How do you present your management plans to patients? There are three distinct categories of skills that you might need here:

- giving people a choice and helping them with their decision
- negotiation skills
- helping patients to feel better before they even leave the room.

Giving patients a choice

It can be helpful to think aloud and be open with patients about your own thoughts and how you've got to this point. If a particular treatment route is not acceptable (for example the request from a parent for antibiotics to deal with a child who has had a runny nose for one day), then you can make this clear. When there are choices (and there almost always are), then tell the patient what these are. Even if there is only one obvious choice, there is almost always a choice to do nothing at all. But often there are quite a number of alternatives:

- do nothing and wait to see what happens
- home remedies
- continue what the patient has already been doing
- come back in a pre-agreed time for review
- an investigation (blood test, X-ray, etc)
- a prescription of some sort
- referral to some one else
    - a doctor or nurse in the practice with a special interest
    - another health professional such as a physiotherapist, podiatrist
    - hospital consultant
- hospital admission.

It is, of course, unhelpful to merely list the choices and ask the patient to pick one of them: 'Do you want to do nothing, have a prescription, a referral to Dr Bloggs or come back and see me next week?' is very likely to be met with the answer:

- 'Well, what do you think, doctor...?' OR
- 'You're the doctor/nurse – you tell me!' (the irritation here is entirely under-standable).

So, in order to give patients a real choice, you have to give them enough information to be able to make a safe, sensible and informed decision. For example, explain:

- what will happen if they do nothing (will they get better in a week or two or could doing nothing lead to significant risks or problems?)

- what the advantages and possible side effects of drug treatment might be
- what tests you might do and why
- what a hospital consultant might do, how long this might take and what advantage, if any, would it offer over managing the problem in primary care.

If you explain your thoughts clearly, it will encourage the patient to do the same, so you can then have a more open and adult discussion about what to do.

Ethics of choice

GP registrars, learning how to consult, can be very unsure about whether it is ethical or professional to offer alternatives and choice when there is 'only one' treatment. An example here is the patient you diagnose with a chest infection for which you would normally prescribe an antibiotic. Is it reasonable to offer the patient a choice? In offering the alternatives in a meaningful way, you need to explain the advantages and disadvantages of each and it is, of course, fine to give the patient your opinion.

> 'What I would generally do for a patient who, like you, was unwell, had a productive cough for more than a week and where I could hear signs of infection in the chest, would be to prescribe a course of .... This would tend to put things right more quickly than doing nothing and avoid the small possibility of the infection getting worse.'

You could then go into the alternative options.

> 'We could do nothing and it's very likely that it would get better on its own, but it might take longer. You could certainly continue with paracetamol and cough medicine, and this would help you to feel better whilst your body makes the antibodies to fight off the infection.
>   A further alternative would be to give you a prescription for antibiotics, but have you hold onto it for the moment. If, over the next few days, you weren't getting any better (or felt worse), then you could take the script to the chemist and get started on the antibiotics.'

You could then check this out with the patient: 'What are your thoughts at the moment?' Given access to the sort of information on which you have based your thinking, many patients will choose the same course of action as you. Those who choose a different course of action, or nothing, would almost certainly not have complied with the treatment had you imposed it on them. Letting them into your thinking process means that you are treating them as adults, empowering them about decisions related to their own health, educating them and allowing them to be more in control. It is, of course, good practice to keep notes on why a particular treatment decision has been reached.

> 'Suggested antibiotics but patient declined these at the moment. Prefers to wait and see – will return for further consultation if cough worse/more systemically unwell over next 2–3 days.'

Should you always offer patients a choice?

There are some situations where it's difficult to think of reasonable alternatives, for example for a 45-year-old woman who has found a breast lump that feels suspicious. It would be difficult for most clinicians to offer a series of reasonable options here, although there may well be choice in terms of *where* to make the urgent referral. In these circumstances, it is very useful to have already found out (by asking!) what thoughts the patient has had. It may be helpful to state: 'I think we need to get this checked out as soon as possible. How does that sound to you?' You can then offer choices about NHS or private, St Elsewhere's or the local hospital, etc.

Each of us has our own comfort zone within which we feel OK offering choices. This will vary between clinicians and some will offer patients a choice in circumstances where others would be more prescriptive. Quite clearly there are some situations where you just get on and treat someone regardless, without offering choices – so if I have a cardiac arrest in front of you, don't waste time offering me the options of being resuscitated or not – just get on with it, please!

Negotiation skills

There are times when, although there are several courses of action or choices to be made, you would actually like to be able to persuade or influence someone in a particular direction. Occasionally you can get away with being quite direct.

- 'My own view is that you should definitely ...'
- 'What I would strongly recommend is ...'
- 'You really must ...'

Michael Balint described this as the apostolic function of the doctor; in other words, some patients will do what you say simply because it's you that says it and they have respect for your expertise and charisma. At other times some tools and skills can be useful.

Phrasing information as questions

There are times when you want to make fairly strong statements to patients, but instead of confronting them you can turn what you want to say into a question.

- 'I think you drink too much' becomes 'Have you ever wondered if you drink too much?'
- 'You must lose weight' becomes 'Have you tried anything so far to help you to lose weight?'
- 'Your glycaemic control is terrible' becomes 'How do you feel about your latest blood sugars?'
- 'You really should stop smoking' becomes 'When do you think you'll be able to stop smoking?'. This can open a dialogue and it also incorporates a presupposition that the patient will stop smoking at some point, which alone can be influential.

The above *statements* might well:

- be received with resistance
- make the patient feel threatened
- provoke a 'stone wall' response.

As *questions* they:

- are softer and less confrontational
- need an answer of some sort and so open the route to a dialogue
- give the patient an implicit power to choose, and so
- empower the patient to make choices about their health.

Reframing

What's in a frame? A frame is something we put around a picture, photograph or mirror to 'contain' it. The frame can also be attractive in its own right. In the same way, patients and doctors put frames (or fences) around problems, illnesses or difficulties in order to contain them and make them manageable so they don't spill out all over the place. Sometimes in life, as in art, the frame is also an 'attractive' or 'desirable' thing to have – or an excuse that leads to secondary gain.

- 'I'm a martyr to my migraines.'
- 'I have myalgic encephalomyelitis (ME) – I can't do anything.'
- 'I'm a cancer victim.'

Do you remember how Tom Sawyer got his friends to paint the fence for him? It was a Saturday morning and he was desperate to enjoy the freedom and sunshine of the day. Painting the fence was a terrible chore and seemed endlessly long. There were several ways that he could have coped with this:

- gritted his teeth and got on with it
- grumbled to his friends about how awful it all was
- pleaded with his friends to help him.

He tries several strategies:

- negotiation – he sees a friend carrying buckets of water and offers to share that chore in return for some help with the whitewashing; the friend declines
- bribery – he offers the friend a marble and a peek at his sore toe; the friend is tempted, particularly by the sore toe, but feels that he shouldn't get involved.

So none of these strategies works and they don't get him the outcome he wanted. Instead, he reframed the problem. He took as his starting point the outrageous and highly unlikely supposition that painting the fence was a rare treat, a skilful task that was a privilege and not something that just anyone could do.

> 'Like it? Well I don't see why I oughtn't to like it. Does a boy get a chance to whitewash a fence every day?'

Before long, his friends were all begging him to let them help and even paying him for the privilege! Tom gains:

- an afternoon off
- a fence that has three coats of whitewash
- 12 marbles, a tin soldier, a kitten with one eye, a dog collar and other goodies.

Reframing can be a really useful skill in helping patients to change their behaviours and a very helpful way of enabling them to come to terms with distressing problems or diagnoses.

> 'I can't sleep, doctor. It's terrible, I'm awake tossing and turning all night. Why can't I have something to help me sleep, it's really awful. Can't you give me some of those temazepam like old Dr Smith used to?'

This is a common enough consultation that can be dealt with in several ways. But after you have tried reassurance, exploration of possible depression and sleep hygiene advice and nothing has worked, what do you do next? It can lead to an impasse where the patient is adamant that they want sleeping tablets and you either refuse or give in. Instead of an argument, you can reframe the situation.

> 'You know, you are so lucky that your body only needs a little sleep. Think of all those extra hours of living that you have compared with everyone else. You don't have to waste your life sleeping like some other unfortunate people. You have an extra 3 or 4 hours every single day of your life – you could take up a new hobby, read those books no one else has time to or do a degree course. I really envy you!'

Of course, this can fall on stony ground and some patients won't respond to it, but many patients will accept this as a reframe. The 'problem' is turned into an opportunity. 'I can't sleep' becomes 'I have more wakeful hours'. The misfortune of being unable to sleep is turned into the advantage of extra life. Instead of being unlucky that they can't sleep well, they are fortunate to have such a wakeful body.

Some cases are more difficult than insomnia, but you can use the same skills even in more difficult and tragic situations.

Example

Alice, a 60-year-old widow, thought she was cured of her breast cancer as she had been clear of it for 10 years. It resurfaced and she was devastated to learn that it was in her bones and her liver. Initially, she was utterly distraught at the thought of 'so little time left'. I saw her each week at the surgery and when it became clear that the initial shock and devastation were wearing off, helped her to explore the things that she would really like to do:

- get her affairs in order
- revisit the island where she and her husband had honeymooned
- take her grandson to Paris
- buy some red shoes.

The stark reality of 'so little time left' was reframed into 'time to focus on what is really important.'

Other ways of giving information

Of course, as well as giving information to patients verbally you can also give them written information or even an audiotape. Some practice computer systems allow you to access Mentor or similar programmes and through this you can print off personalised information leaflets. This is an excellent way of reinforcing what you have said.

Possible action points

- Video record one of your surgeries and watch it alone or with a colleague. What skills do you use when you are giving information to patients? Are there any skills that you don't use at the moment that you could usefully add to your toolkit?

- Pay attention to the patient's vocabulary of nouns, verbs and representational states. Practise incorporating these into your information-giving.
- 'Eliminate the negative, accentuate the positive!' as the words of the song go. Get into the habit of phrasing statements positively. It can feel difficult or unnatural at first, but comes much more easily with practice.

Further reading

- Balint M. *The Doctor, his Patient and the Illness*. London: Pitman Medical; 1957. 2nd edn Edinburgh: Churchill Livingstone; 1964, reprinted 1986.
- Neighbour R. *The Inner Consultation*. Lancaster: MTP Press; 1987. 2nd edn Oxford: Radcliffe Publishing; 2004.
- Silverman J, Kurtz S, Draper J. *Skills for Communicating with Patients*. Oxford: Radcliffe Medical Press; 1998. 2nd edn; 2004.

Chapter 10

Safety-netting and ending

The sky is darkening like a stain
Something is going to fall like rain
And it won't be flowers.

'The Witnesses', WH Auden*

Key points

- Safety-netting is a very important phase of most consultations and can help to empower patients as well as protect doctors, nurses and other health professionals.
- It is not enough to say 'Come back if you are no better'.
- Safety-netting is essential in all consultations where you are working with limited information.
- Good endings help patients to feel better as they leave the room.

Safety-netting is a very useful way to draw consultations to a close and it is another tool that helps empower patients about their management. Many consultations include some sort of rather loose safety net and, when videoed, the clinician's last words to the patient are often something like, 'Come back if you're no better'. And the patient often smiles or nods and goes out of the room. The doctor or nurse also smiles and mentally ticks off 'safety-netted' and knows that they will be in the clear if something goes wrong and can sleep peacefully in their bed tonight. They may even write in the medical record: 'TRIN' (to return if necessary), 'Scc if not settling' or 'See as required'.

Unfortunately this is more like a leaky sieve than a safety net and is full of holes that the patient might just fall through. If you think back (or refer now) to Chapter 5, you will realise that this phrase is well-meant but full of generalisations.

- 'Come back.' Come back where? Here? To see this clinician? Or would anyone do? When should I come back? Today? Tomorrow? In a year? Now???
- 'If you're no better.' No better when? In 5 minutes, a week, a month? How long will it take? How would I know that I'm no better? What's the time scale of this illness anyway?

And come to that, if I do come back, what is going to happen? Is this likely to be something serious or is it quite trivial?

The primary care problem

The challenge of primary care, as my first trainer said to me many years ago, is that of 20 patients you see in a morning surgery, 19 will have something trivial wrong with them so it doesn't matter very much what you do or don't do, so long

---

*Reprinted with permission of Faber and Faber Ltd from *Collected Poems* by WH Auden.

as you don't actively harm them. The 20th patient will have something really wrong with them and the dilemma is working out which one is that patient. Anyone who has worked in primary care for any length of time will have their own personal examples of the following:

- the baby with a runny nose who was admitted later with epiglottitis
- the child with anxious parents and a mild viral illness who was rushed to A&E the same evening with meningococcal meningitis
- the telephone consultation with an anxious young man with left elbow pain that you were sure was musculoskeletal, who had a cardiac arrest within the hour (and was successfully resuscitated only because someone with the right equipment was, by chance, in the right place at the right time)
- the depressed woman who definitely didn't have suicidal ideation when you asked her, but who jumped to her death under an express train later the same day.

Primary care can be a jungle of deception. We see patients early in their illnesses, particularly now that there is advanced access and they really can get an appointment today. We can be lulled into a false security by the fact that most patients have self-limiting illnesses and that common things are common. We have 10 minutes for each patient to make a decision and get it right – and the consequences of being wrong can be devastating for everyone.

Using a safety net is an essential protection for both patient and clinician and, used well, should ensure that neither of you falls too far.

Effective safety nets

A proper safety net will catch the patient so that they don't fall through the holes. Neighbour (1987) describes a very effective three-part safety net.

1. **Tell the patient what you think is wrong and what you expect to happen**
   'I think this is likely to be viral and you should be feeling a lot better by the weekend.'
2. **How the *patient* would know if you're wrong**
   'If it's going on longer than 10 days or so, and particularly if you start to feel worse in yourself or start coughing a lot of stuff up ...'
3. **What they should do then**
   'Come back and see me and I'll have another listen to your chest/arrange an X-ray/get you seen at the hospital.'

Safety-netting is a really useful tool in all consultations but is essential in any consultation where you have less information than usual, for example:

- telephone consultations, where you have no visual cues
- out-of-hours consultations, where you have no previous knowledge of the patient.

If you find yourself having to consult when you are tired or not up to your usual form, for any reason, then make sure the consultation has a watertight safety net.

Ending consultations

By this point, the consultation is drawing to a close. As well as a safety net, there are several other aspects to consider.

- **Discussing if or when you will see the patient again**
  'Book an appointment with me in 2 weeks so I can see how you are doing.'
  'I'll leave it with you – we should probably touch base in the next few weeks.'
- **A final summary**
  'So just to recap – stay off work for the next week, make sure you take the antibiotics three times a day and come back in a week if you aren't nearly back to normal then.'
- **A final check**
  'Is there anything that isn't clear or you would like me to recap?'
- **A catch-all**
  'Was there anything else at all?'

The catch-all is both wonderful and dangerous! As the patient (and I speak from experience) it feels as if the clinician both cares whether there is something that you have not yet dared to say and is willing to deal with it. As the clinician, it sometimes uncovers patients' problems that are really significant and that they are immensely relieved to tell you, and this is very satisfying. It's also dangerous because you can't say it without genuinely having the time and willingness to deal with whatever the patient says, even if all you do is listen enough to negotiate a further consultation soon. However good your skills, there will be some patients who save the 'real' problem to the end, not because they're being awkward or obstructive, but because this is the only way that they can tell you at all. Use it if you can; try it out when you aren't too busy or under time pressure.

Good endings

When the consultation ends well, the patient will leave the room well on the way to feeling better. Of course, the ending is only as good as what has preceded it but, assuming that the rest of the consultation has been good enough, the following will help ensure a good ending:

- maintaining rapport with the patient
- being as sure as you can that you have dealt with the patient's problems appropriately, and that the communication and process of consultation have gone well enough so far
- being alert to the possibility of a last-minute disclosure and allowing space for this
- not rushing the patient at the end
- ending with a warm smile and a few words such as 'Take care now', 'Look after yourself', 'Thank you for coming to see me'.

Possible action points

- Watch a video of your consultations and note what your current pattern of safety-netting is. How often do you use a safety net? Is it an adequate net or one with holes in it?
- Practise using a 3-point safety net in all your consultations.

- Think about how you end consultations; watch what you do on video and consider whether you need to do anything differently.
- If you don't generally say 'And was there anything else?', give it a try!

References and further reading

- Neighbour R. *The Inner Consultation*. Lancaster: MTP Press; 1987. 2nd edn Oxford: Radcliffe Publishing; 2004.
- Silverman J, Kurtz S, Draper J. *Skills for Communicating with Patients*. Oxford: Radcliffe Medical Press; 1998. 2nd edn; 2004.

Chapter 11

Managing time

Tomorrow, and tomorrow, and tomorrow,
Creeps in this petty pace from day to day,
To the last syllable of recorded time;
And all our yesterdays have lighted fools
The way to dusty death. Out, out, brief candle!
Life's but a walking shadow; a poor player,
That struts and frets his hour upon the stage,
And then is heard no more: it is a tale
Told by an idiot, full of sound and fury,
Signifying nothing.

Macbeth, William Shakespeare

Key points

- Managing time effectively and efficiently is one of the keys to good consultations — for both doctor and patient.
- It is very difficult to have an adequate consultation that lasts less than 10 minutes.
- Most patients have no idea (unless you tell them) how long a consultation is booked for.
- A great deal can be accomplished in 10 minutes — and even more if both doctor and patient are clear about the time boundaries.
- Some consultations will inevitably run on longer than this, no matter how skilled you are.
- Using some of the techniques in this book will help you to make your consultations more time-efficient.
- Keeping to time matters much more to some people than others.
- You can learn both to manage time more effectively in the consultation and also to get less stressed when you do run late.

How long is your consultation?

There's a short answer and a longer answer! Of course, the easy way is to look at your consultation booking intervals – 5 minutes, 7.5 minutes, 10 minutes, 15 minutes or even longer and think about whether you tend to finish on time, are generally running late or find yourself with spare time between consultations. But this doesn't tell the full picture. To work out how long your consultation really is, you need to think about the following questions as well.

Do you generally start on time?

Or do you arrive in your room at the allotted time and then switch on the computer and printer (2 minutes), then go and make a cup of coffee (3 minutes), check your post or email (5 minutes) and then call the first patient, now anything up to 10 minutes late.

How long do you actually spend with the patient?

This will be less than your consultation interval. Depending on how you summon patients, it may take a minute or more for them to get to your room. At the end of the consultation, it may take a minute or two to type up the consultation. That 10-minute consultation has actually been reduced to 7 minutes or less. If you spend 2 minutes whilst the patient is with you entering data on the computer and tidying up the drug record, you may be down to 5 minutes of real contact with the patient.

Do you finish on time?

Some clinicians finish their surgeries promptly most of the time, but others regularly finish 20–30 minutes late or even later than that. Those 10-minute appointments may actually be 15 minutes long on average, with a clinician who may or may not get stressed about the fact that they invariably finish later than their colleagues, who themselves may or may not be stressed about the fact that Dr A or Nurse B is never there for coffee or when the visits are being shared out.

So what's 'normal'?

Doctors and nurses consult at a whole range of intervals, most commonly between 5 and 15 minutes, with an average of 7½ to 10 minutes. The 'norm' for doctors in training, and training practices, is to consult at 10-minute intervals. This consultation interval also attracts quality points and payments within the new GMS contract.

With the increasing complexity of consultations (health promotion, collecting data for targets, reviews of medication, etc) it is likely that more consultations need to last for a longer, rather than a shorter, period of time. I suspect that within the next 5 years (10 at the most) the 15-minute consultation will be normal.

Do your patients know how long their consultation is?

This is so obvious to any doctor, nurse or their reception staff that we often forget that it isn't equally clear to patients. When a patient books an appointment, they are almost always told that the appointment is at 8.30 or 10.50 am, or whatever. So they are told the starting time, but not that the appointment is from 8.30 to 8.40 am or from 10.50 to 10.55 am.

If patients are clearer about consultation length, then they can often work out how to manage the time and are less likely to come in with an unrealistic expectation of how much can be fitted into a single appointment.

> **Example**
>
> A number of years ago, I worked for a Health Authority supporting small practices and was asked to do a locum surgery in an inner-city practice in a

deprived area. Knowing that appointments at this surgery tended to be short and anticipating that the patients might have significant health needs, I specifically asked for the patients to be booked for my surgery at 10-minute intervals. When I arrived, I was horrified to find that patients were booked at 5-minute intervals for the next 2 hours — a total of 24 patients scheduled to begin at 4 pm and end at 6 pm. I envisaged a very long surgery going on until at least 8 pm or even later. To my amazement, the patients all came in with '5-minute problems'. They had all learnt through experience over the years that they had a 5-minute consultation and almost every one of them came in with a very brief, well-defined problem that could, at least superficially, be dealt with in the time available. Of course, sorting out their underlying problems would have taken very much longer.

Time management problems

When doctors or nurses talk about difficulties they have with keeping to time or managing time effectively in the consultation, there tend to be a number of common themes:

- they always run late and feel stressed about this
- they have trouble with ending the consultation in a satisfactory way
- just as they think they've finished the consultation, the patient comes out with another problem, and then another
- they feel obliged to deal with all the problems that the patient presents during the consultation, even if there are several and they are already running behind
- they find it hard to get some patients to shut up
- they can't get patients out of the door.

What do you tell the patients when you are running late?

Most patients accept that sometimes other people's consultations last longer than they should and that at times they may be kept waiting. Giving people timely information and choice can make a difference to how the consultation will run.

In some practices, reception staff will be alert to the fact that you are running well over time and will spontaneously say this to the patients. For example:

- telling patients who are already in the waiting room that you are running late and that they will be seen, but later than booked
- saying the same thing to patients who book in at the desk
- offering patients a choice about whether to wait or rebook (or any other options, such as a consultation with another health professional who is less busy).

When patients come into your room you can, of course, say nothing and just get on with the consultation, but quite often patients are somewhat irritated or annoyed. Sometimes this comes out directly:

- 'You're running late today.'
- 'I nearly had to go — I've been waiting so long.'
- 'I've got to be somewhere else in 10 minutes.'

At other times this is not expressed verbally and directly, but can manifest itself either as irritated behaviour or an active 'go slow', with patients appearing to 'dare' you to not deal with their list of six problems, today – yes, all of them. So a brief, bland but sincere acknowledgement that you have kept them waiting can be very helpful:

- 'Sorry you've had to wait'
- 'Sorry I'm running behind today'.

This is usually enough to defuse any irritation or anger, and help you and the patient to get on with what they are there for.

When patients are late

In most practices, I suspect that clinicians are much later than patients, who tend to be there on time for their appointments!

Early in my career, when I had a very misplaced sense of self-importance, I used to get stressed if patients kept me waiting for more than a few minutes, particularly if they didn't offer some sort of explanation or apology when they eventually got into the consulting room. I even used to get cross if I realised from the timings on the computer that the patient had arrived a bit late even when I was already running behind. It didn't take me long to learn that saying something at the beginning of the consultation (any variant on 'You're late') immediately interfered with the rest of the consultation and sometimes completely ruined it. So I used to grit my teeth and hang onto the irritation until the end of the consultation when I would say something like, 'Were you held up today?' or 'By the way — can I just mention that you were late today and I was waiting for you'. By the end of the consultation, the patient had usually completely forgotten that they had been late in the first place and the reminder sometimes came as an unpleasant surprise and an extremely poor ending to the consultation for both of us.

When I realised how stressed this made me, never mind the patients, feel, I made a conscious decision to be more relaxed about patients' punctuality. After all, few patients set out with the intention of being late and I know I keep my patients waiting, on average, far longer than they ever make me wait for them. My stress disappeared completely with this reframing.

Timelines

So why do some health professionals get very stressed about time in the consultation when others don't? The concept of 'timelines' can help to explain this. Spend a few moments thinking about what has happened in your past. Focus on a significant event. Point towards it. Where is it located (behind/in front/to the left/to the right)? Now think about your future, something you would really like to do. Where is this located? Point to it. Now imagine a line that connects your past to your future — this is called your timeline.

NLP suggests that some people are 'in time' and others are 'through time'. Those who are 'in time' usually have their timeline running from front to back. Their past is literally behind them and their future is ahead. These people live in the 'now' part of the timeline. They are less aware of the passage of time and are more spontaneous. They may find it difficult to meet deadlines and be punctual. Their consultations may run late, but it doesn't usually worry them. On the other hand, people who are 'through time' have the past, present and future in front of them. Usually their timeline runs from left to right. These people are punctual and good planners but may tend to get stressed when consultations over-run.

So do you always run late or are you punctual or mostly punctual? If you do run late, is this something that you want to change? Does it cause you or your patients to be stressed?

Possible action points

- If time causes you problems in the consultation, consider what steps you could take to reduce your stress in this area.
- If your consultation booking interval is currently less than 10 minutes, it is worth thinking about changing it to 10 minutes. It is nearly impossible to have a good consultation in anything less and, even if you have an adequate consultation, it is quite likely that patients will return with unfinished business within a short space of time. If you work in a partnership where the norm is to have less than 10 minutes for an appointment, this may need some negotiation and clearly you may need to have longer surgeries in order to see the same number of patients as colleagues who choose to consult more rapidly. Some doctors who have tried this find that they may have an apparently longer surgery than their partners, but in fact they finish at the same time that they have been finishing anyway, only now they end on time rather than being half an hour late and it is all much less stressful!
- Tell patients how long their consultation with you is. You could do this by putting a poster up in the waiting room ('Consultations last 10 minutes') or by asking your staff to tell patients when they book: 'Your appointment is from 9 o'clock to 10 past 9 with Dr X'. Patients will soon get the hang of this and learn the length of their consultation.
- Make sure you start on time. If you are a perpetual 'only just in time' person, you may need to plan to arrive 15 minutes earlier than normal to achieve this.
- Learn to recognise the patient cues that suggest that there is more than one problem to be dealt with and get this out in the open as early as you can.
- Practise strategies for dealing with patients with 'lists'.
- Practise breaking rapport as a way of getting reluctant patients to end consultations.
- Learn to touch-type if you can't do this at the moment or invest in voice recognition software.
- Make sure patients know that they can book a longer appointment (e.g. 20 minutes) if they wish.
- Practise a brief, bland form of words that apologises to patients if you have kept them waiting — enough to deal with their frustration, but not so much that it crowds out their opening.

Further reading

- O'Connor J, McDermott I. *Principles of NLP*. London: Thorsons; 1996.

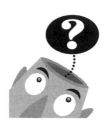

Chapter 12

Transactions in consultations

Key points

- The consultation is a 'transaction' between two individuals.
- At any point in the consultation, health professional and patient can be in any of three different ego states: parent, adult or child.
- The natural role of the health professional is as carer and generally patients are feeling vulnerable when they come and see us so the behaviour pattern of doctor or nurse as caring parent and patient as child is not uncommon.
- A healthier model of the consultation for both health professional and patient is that of two adults.

Eric Berne (1970) described an interesting model of the human psyche that is very useful in primary care consultations. According to Berne, the human psyche has three different states and each of us has all three, moving between them according to the situation in which we find ourselves. The three states are Parent, Adult and Child and at any given point in the consultation (as in any encounter between two individuals) the doctor and the patient are in one of the three ego states. The terms parent, adult and child refer to ways of behaving, not chronological age or parenthood or lack of this.

Child ego state

This refers to behaving, thinking and feeling in ways that were learnt in childhood. Typically, the child ego state is impulsive, instinctive, emotional and full of feelings. Sulking and bad temper may also be present. Three different types of child ego state are described:

- free child – spontaneous and creative
- adapted (hurt) child – whining, manipulative
- little professor – a 'know-all'.

Adult ego state

The adult ego state is the one that deals with complex information and makes effective decisions for living in the world. For example, when driving a car in the rush hour, each of us needs to absorb, assimilate and process an enormous amount of information such as the speed of other cars, pedestrians, cyclists, traffic lights and signals, speed limits, weather conditions. Despite all this, we generally arrive safely at our destination.

The adult ego state also regulates the activities of an individual's 'parent' and 'child', and negotiates some of the decisions between them.

Example

The middle-aged, intermediate skier standing at the top of a difficult run, wondering whether or not to tackle it, may well have internal conversations something like this:

> **Child:** Black run – exciting! I could go really fast down here. Let's go!
>
> **Parent:** Hang on. This is icy – could be dangerous. What's going to happen if you fall and injure your knee? You're not as young as you used to be! That would be the end of your skiing days. You could always side-slip down. There's no shame in that and at least you'll get there in one piece and not on the blood-wagon.
>
> **Adult:** OK. First section looks tricky – could side-slip as far as the first marker pole. Not too bad after that – need to do short turns though. Let's just take it at a steady pace. Check behind for boy-racers – is it clear? Off we go then!

Here the adult ego state has objectively mediated between the impulsive, but reckless, child and the over-cautious, but caring, parent and has balanced the risks.

One really useful function of the adult ego state is that it lets us make many everyday trivial decisions almost automatically and without really thinking about them. This saves time and energy and frees up capacity in our decision-making processes, so that they can be saved for significant and important decisions. The adult ego state helps us make these no-brain decisions quickly so that creative power and energy are freed up for more challenging areas, in other words where they're really needed. If I spend 10 minutes, half a dozen times a day, deciding whether to have tea, coffee, de-caf, herbal, water or nothing at all to drink, then I won't have much time or creative energy left to consult with patients.

Parent ego state

The parent ego state includes caring and nurturing – looking after ourselves and others. It also includes being critical and punishing. It is described as a 'borrowed' ego state; a person in the parental ego state uses ways of thinking, feeling and behaving that are borrowed and copied from parents and parental figures in the past.

How the theory links with general practice consultations

Both doctor and patient are in particular ego states at every moment of the consultation. Patients are often worried, anxious or asking for something when they come to see a doctor and this can sometimes tend to mean that the child ego state dominates. This can have a reciprocal effect on the doctor, whose natural role anyway is often more parent than adult. If doctor and patient had met each other at a social event or in the street they might well each have behaved in adult roles (an adult to adult transaction).

> **Person 1:** 'Excuse me. Do you happen to know the way to the station?'
> **Person 2**: 'Yes. Turn right at the traffic lights, cross the road and it's about 100 metres on the left.'

But put the same two people into a consultation setting and the one who is now the patient can become more childlike and the one who is now the doctor can become more parental.

> **Patient:** 'I'm really worried about this cough – I'm terrified I've got cancer.'
> **Doctor:** 'Don't worry – it's only a chest infection. These antibiotics will make it better.'

Because the natural role of the clinician is to be caring and helpful (usually, at least), the doctor–patient or nurse–patient transactions can sometimes be more parent–child rather than adult–adult. This is not always in the best interests of either of them and can lead to all sorts of problems.

Clinician

The clinician may experience problems such as:

*   burnout or exhaustion through constantly trying to 'make it better' when they can't
*   a sense of failure when things go wrong
*   a set of very needy and emotionally draining patients, who visit regularly.

Patient

The patient may:

*   depend on the doctor
*   fail to take proper responsibility for their own health
*   never get better, because they enjoy the parental-type attention they get when they are 'ill'
*   blame the doctor for failing when they don't get better or things go wrong.

Being familiar with the concepts of Transactional Analysis and one's own behaviour patterns in consultations can be very useful. It can help to identify why consultations go adrift, why some patients keep coming back and never get better, and why some clinicians head for burnout. Increased awareness can help clinicians to break out of unhelpful behaviour patterns and make consultations more flexible, more empowering for patients and more effective.

Possible action points

*   Videos are very helpful here. Video some of your consultations and watch them to see if you can work out which ego state you and the patient are in at particular moments of the consultation.

- Overall, how many of your consultations tend to be in the parent–child pattern and how many are adult–adult?
- If there is a preponderance of parent–child behaviour, what steps could you take to adopt a more adult–adult model?

Reference and further reading

- Berne E. *Games People Play: the psychology of human relationships.* London: Penguin Books Ltd; 1970.

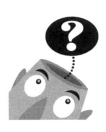

Chapter 13

You, the patient and the computer

'I know that you and Frank were planning to disconnect me, and I'm afraid that's something I cannot allow to happen.'

HAL, the computer, in '2001 A Space Odyssey'

Key points

- Computers are now an almost integral part of the consultation process.
- Any clinicians who learnt most of their consultation skills before the widespread use of computers may well need to adapt them in order to have effective triadic consultations.
- Keyboard and mouse skills, and the ability to touch-type will all help enhance the process of the consultation.
- Try to pay full attention to the patient whenever they are speaking. This may well mean that you stop typing or looking something up and instead turn to the patient.

Like them or loathe them, computers in the consulting room are here to stay. The presence of the computer does, inevitably, have some effect on the consultation and this is a variant on the triadic or three-way consultation. One of the three parties has a fairly passive role and communicates only through the visual medium – it is there, but it doesn't speak.

Clinicians use computer systems in a variety of different ways from very little to totally digital and paper-light. So how do you use the computer in your consultation? It is likely to be in one of the following ways:

1. not at all; the computer is switched off
2. not at all; the computer is switched on but not used
3. only when the patient is out of the room, for example to check the appointments list, call the next patient or enter data
4. to produce a prescription
5. to access information from the patient's record during the consultation, for example to look at results or hospital letters, or to read the notes that you or the last doctor or nurse made
6. to enter information about the consultation, i.e. making notes as you go along
7. to remind you to act on something that needs to be recorded, for example the patient's blood pressure that hasn't been noted for the last year or so, or a smear that is overdue
8. to get information from local or remote databases to enable decision making, for example to check Medline, Prodigy or other sources of information
9. as information sources for the patient, for patient education or as a data source for shared decision-making.

As computers are used more and more in the consultation, and keeping good records of data is essential for quality points and so forth, the real challenge is in being able to make the process of the consultation as effective as possible at the same time as using the computer. Some of this will depend on how confident you are at using the computer and how good you are at multitasking – being an effective juggler and doing more than one thing at once. It will be easier if, like driving a car, you are unconsciously competent with the computer. If you are still at the conscious competence stage, or even conscious incompetence, it will be more challenging.

But however skilful you are with the keyboard and mouse, it is difficult (or impossible) to give your full attention to both the patient and the computer screen at the same time. It's also important to be aware that the patient may say something really significant or important when your own attention is directed mainly at the computer screen.

Improving consultations involving the computer

Consider rearranging your desk

Some clinicians have the screen turned so that only they can read it. This can feel very secretive and intimidating to the patient, who may spend at least part of the consultation wondering or worrying about what you are writing about them. Having the computer as a tool that is shared by both clinician and patient can help to deal with this.

If you want to give this a go, try sitting in the patient's chair in your room and look at the computer screen. Is it legible? Is the light reflecting on it so that nothing can be read? Move the screen until both clinician and patient can see it clearly.

Use signposting

Signpost what you are doing so that the patient knows when you are attending to them and when you are attending to the computer's needs. In other words express clearly to the patient that, for a few moments, they will not have your full attention.

- 'I'm just going to look at the computer now.'
- 'Hang on a sec whilst I just have a look at EMIS/TOREX.'
- 'You'll have to bear with me. I'm still learning how to use these computers/touch type.'

This is much more effective than trying to do two things at once or, equally, not telling the patient what you are doing. Just turning away from them to attend to the computer can be perceived by the patient as lack of interest or attention, or just plain rude.

Instead, make it as clear as you can to the patient when you are really listening to them and they have your full attention (i.e. by facing them, making eye contact, being in rapport, non-verbally communicating etc) and when you are entering or looking up information on the computer.

Another way of attempting to ensure that significant information is confined to the time that the patient has your full attention is to use small talk whenever you are looking at the screen. This will help to fill the gap and avoid space for the patient to disclose. Small talk will consist of whatever you can talk about without thinking too much (for example the weather, holidays, EastEnders, the football etc). If the patient does start talking when you are looking at the screen, immediately stop what you are doing and turn your full attention back to them.

Share information from the computer with the patient

There may well be information on the computer that you can or wish to share with the patient. How much of this you do will be determined by your attitude towards sharing information with patients in general and involving patients in the decision-making process. If there is a whole screen of text, you might need to point out the relevant section. Do give the patient the opportunity to ask questions.

Possible action points

- Experiment with the computer turned towards the patient as a shared tool.
- Practise signposting what you are doing, and attending to the patient or the computer at any one moment but not both together.
- If your typing skills are getting in the way, go on a touch-typing course. This could be part of your personal learning plan.
- You could even invest in voice-recognition software.

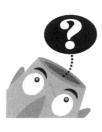

Chapter 14

Looking after yourself

Energy can be changed from one form to another, but it cannot be created or destroyed. The total amount of energy and matter in the Universe remains constant, merely changing from one form to another.

(First Law of Thermodynamics)

Key points

- Consultations are stressful and emotionally draining.
- You are the key diagnostic and therapeutic tool in the consultation and it is vital to keep yourself in good shape.
- It is important to have a range of ways of looking after yourself between consultations, day to day, medium term and long term.

'Housekeeping' is a term first coined by Neighbour (1987) but now fully assimilated into consultation-skills language. It refers to a part of the consultation that is sometimes left out altogether and certainly one that often isn't given its full attention.

Think for a moment about one of those really awful consultations that has got your heart racing and your blood churning, and the patient has just walked out clearly angry, distressed or dissatisfied. In all likelihood, this consultation ran well over its allotted time so that as well as being stressed you are also now running late. What would you do now?

- Do you call in the next patient, grit your teeth and get on with it?
- Do you have any way of letting off steam before the next consultation?
- If you are already running late (and awful consultations often seem to last longer than their allotted time), does it just add to your stress to take a break of any sort? After all, you'll run even later if you do!

What about at the end of surgery? You've seen 16 patients in an ordinary surgery (on a good day, if you're lucky), or maybe you've seen 24 patients or even more. Some, if not all, of these consultations will have involved you giving something of yourself. After all, this is why patients come to see us; we are not machines or interactive computer programmes but real people with our own feelings, strengths, weaknesses and vulnerabilities, which we bring to the process of the consultation. Our own emotions play a greater or lesser part in each consultation and seeing patients is stressful. As well as giving of yourself, it is very likely that you will also have received from the patient. Think about the patient who came in distressed, angry, confused or anxious and who walks out looking much better and thanking you sincerely for helping them. What has happened to all those feelings and all the energy surrounding them? One of the fundamental laws of physics states that energy and matter can neither be created nor destroyed and the same is true for emotional energy. It may be transformed — perhaps from tears to laughter — but often it is simply transmitted from the patient to the clinician. The patient feels better and the clinician, who has another dozen patients left to see, just absorbs it.

So what about the end of the week, or after a month or three? Forty patient interactions a day (and that's a fairly low tally — some doctors or nurses will have a hundred consultations, visits, telephone calls, etc) is 200 in a week — nearly a thousand a month. That's a lot of consultations and uses up a lot of inner resources.

The process of consultation requires you to:

- actively listen to a complex story and make some sense of it
- recognise whether you are dealing with something trivial or something that is so significant that it needs immediate attention
- in the course of a single hour, see patients:
    - of all ages from birth to 100+
    - who are pregnant, dying, anxious, worried or well, etc
    - who have a complex entanglement of physical, emotional and psychosocial illness
- shift your emotions every 10 minutes so that, for example, you can helpfully manage an infertile patient when you have just referred the previous patient for a termination of an unwanted pregnancy (or vice versa)
- diagnose and prescribe appropriately, remembering all the potential drug interactions
- manage on-going chronic illnesses
- think about whether there is any information that you require from the patient in order to achieve quality points
- Read code what you are doing
- ... and all of this in 10 minutes.

It is hardly surprising that the process of primary care consultation is stressful to the health professionals who engage in it. After all, the main diagnostic and therapeutic tool used is not the computer programme, the latest NICE guidelines or a clever algorithm about gastro-oesophageal reflux disease (GORD) — it is oneself. The self can take quite a lot of battering along the rollercoaster ride of a surgery. Repeated trauma without paying attention to oneself is a prescription for stress, burnout, depression, alcohol use, marital break up and all the other illnesses to which doctors and other health professionals are prone.

Just as housekeeping is important between consultations (are you *really* ready for the next patient?), it is also important to consolidate this with regular attention to the self on a daily and weekly basis, and long term. Always remember that *you* are the key tool in the consultation. So how do you look after yourself in the short and long term in order to stay in good shape?

Between patients

Housekeeping between consultations means ensuring that you are in a fit state to deal with the next consultation and that you don't have any negative feelings from the last one still hanging around. Sometimes there are so many negative feelings that you can't get rid of them all in just a few minutes of diversion time.

So at times housekeeping is about ensuring that you have dealt with enough of the feelings in the short term, but have a definite plan to come back and deal with the rest at a suitable time very soon.

There are three quick and easy ways to help get rid of negative feelings or stress between patients. These fall broadly into the three categories of kinaesthetic, auditory and visual and you might want to choose one that fits well with your own representational system.

Kinaesthetic methods

These methods of de-stressing work well for most people. After all, the stress is in the kinaesthetic part of you, so it makes sense to pay particular attention to this area in order to help to manage it.

It's likely you have been more or less stuck in your chair during a stressful consultation and your body posture may have become tense. Just physically getting out of the position you were in will help to loosen the muscles and shake out tension. The first thing to do, then, is to get up out of the chair and move around. As well as standing up, you could walk about to distract yourself with something. Some examples might be:

- going to a different part of your room, for example to take a book off the shelf or to wash your hands
- walking to the kitchen to make yourself a cup of coffee or get a glass of water
- going down to reception to see what's happening there
- going outside the building and walking around it.

When you've done this and sat back down in your chair, you might want to do some other physical activity at your desk to help to get you back into a good state for seeing patients, for example:

- checking your email for new messages
- checking for pathology results that may have come through
- reading any hospital letters
- signing a bundle of repeat prescriptions.

Auditory methods

Talking and listening are also good ways of de-stressing between patients. This might be face to face or on the phone. So if, as well as getting up out of your chair and walking somewhere, you also find someone to have a quick conversation with so much the better. This might be:

- a partner or colleague who happens to have a free moment
- the practice nurse
- reception staff.

You could also make that phone call that needs to be fitted in some time this morning or afternoon.

If you are a particularly auditory person, it might well be that you already have some sort of music system set up in your room. Just playing a favourite piece of music for a few minutes and consciously immersing yourself in it can be very therapeutic and a good way of getting rid of stress.

Visual methods

Many health professionals have pictures, photographs or plants in their rooms. Having visual reminders of people or occasions that are special for you can be particularly useful when you are stressed after a consultation. Being able to look at a reminder of, for example, a really good time on holiday or members of your family can help to shift your emotions out of the negative residual feelings that you have and back to more positive ones.

Some doctors or nurses like to have photos of their family — partners and/or children in particular — on their desks. Others don't; some prefer not to have their family on display, others find that it can sometimes be unhelpful when consulting with a patient who has, for instance, marital problems, infertility or a child who has died. But a photograph or picture that has significance for you does not necessarily need to be one that is obvious to anyone else. A picture of a view, for instance, might just look like a pretty picture to anyone else but might link you to the best holiday you ever had or a special moment with family or friends.

Medium term

So the patient has left, you've got yourself back together enough to carry on and see the patients left in the surgery and manage the rest of the day. What can you do this week or next week to deal with this and all the other stresses that you may gather during the rest of the week?

Most practitioners who deal with people's emotional needs on a day-to-day basis, have supervision and support built into their working lives in a way that is rare in medicine. Counsellors, for example, have supervision — a regular debriefing meeting with a professional colleague in which they can explore and offload all aspects of their work with clients and look particularly at the effect clients may be having on them as well as exploring any blind spots that they may, themselves, have with clients. They also usually have personal therapy — an hour a week with a professional counsellor, which is time for themselves. Very, very few GPs or nurses have anything like this!

Regular time built into this week and every week is incredibly helpful in terms of managing stress. Within the practice, you might:

- all meet regularly for coffee and debriefing
- meet for lunch together at least once a week
- have buddying sessions where two of you get together to debrief
- organise your workload so that each of you has either a half or whole day off, or an early finish each week, or both
- have regular educational sessions where you look at consultations, for example through random or problem-case analysis.

If you are single-handed, could you buddy up with someone in a neighbouring practice?

Outside the practice itself, there are other opportunities:

- groups of practitioners that meet on a regular basis can be a really helpful place to debrief and de-stress; these include:
  - study groups such as MRCGP or post-MRCGP groups
  - professional support groups

- personal support groups, possibly with a facilitator
- groups of practitioners, for example young principal groups
- mentoring and co-mentoring relationships.

Many postgraduate centres will have details of local, trained mentors who will be willing to listen and offer space for colleagues to explore issues. This tends to be a one-way relationship and often lasts for a prescribed number of sessions, six being typical.

Co-mentoring can work well too. Here two practitioners agree to meet with each other on a regular basis to offer mutual support. Typically, the time is divided equally so that one listens whilst the other talks and they then swap over. Ideally, you need a like-minded colleague, whose work is similar enough to yours to allow them to fully understand what you do and appreciate any difficulties that it might cause, but who is someone that you don't work with directly on any regular basis. Because this is a two-way relationship, it is more sustainable than one-way mentoring. Some people find the power dynamics of a one-way relationship difficult and this is overcome by co-mentoring, where the relationship is equal and neither party owes anything or has power of any sort over the other.

Balint groups

Balint groups are still popular and are usually run on psychodynamic lines. There are usually two co-facilitators: one is likely to be a psychotherapist, the other may well be a GP who has trained as a Balint facilitator. These groups are a useful forum for doctors to explore blocks or difficulties that are causing problems in consultations. One of Balint's key ideas was that doctors, either consciously or unconsciously, decide what they will allow patients to discuss in the consultation, choosing from the list of problems that the patient brings. Equally, doctors may place restraints and embargoes on certain areas, and again this may well be sub-conscious. This selective neglect or avoidance may be related to something in the doctor's life that feels threatening. For example, a doctor may ignore signals from a patient that there is a marital problem if the doctor also has a similar problem or if they are close to someone else who does. If the patient is reluctant or ambivalent about exploring this issue, this can lead to collusion.

Balint groups traditionally begin with the facilitator asking, 'Has anyone got a case today?' A brave volunteer then tells the story of a bothersome patient and the group tries to help them identify and explore the blocks that are constraining exploration and management of the patient's problem. It should be noted that Balint groups are not therapy groups for clinicians and that the focus is very much on the patient rather than the clinician.

Longer term

Looking after yourself in the long term is about achieving balance in your life. The balancing point is different at various stages of your career and life, but some aspects are important throughout:

- achieving a balance between:
  - time at work and family time
  - money and free time
  - ambition and status quo

- activities outside medicine such as:
  - hobbies
  - music, theatre, cinema
  - sport, recreation, exercise
- relationships with family, friends and colleagues.

Are you where you want to be at the moment? If not, what needs to change? If you are, will you still be in the right place in 5 or 10 years' time?

Possible action points

- Identify ways that you get rid of stress or negative feelings at the moment between patients. Are these effective or do you need to add new ways?
- What do you do each week that helps you to look after yourself? Is this enough? Do you need to amend it in any way?
- Do you have an overall, long-term plan? Is your life in balance? If not, what steps could you take to help achieve this?

References and further reading

- Chambers R. *Survival Skills for GPs.* Oxford: Radcliffe Medical Press; 1999.
- Neighbour R. *The Inner Consultation*. Lancaster: MTP Press; 1987. 2nd edn Oxford: Radcliffe Publishing; 2004.
- www.balint.co.uk

Part 2

Tools and techniques for learning and improving consultation skills

Introduction

This section of the book will help you identify what you might learn and how to go about it. Reflecting on your current practice and learning new skills will not only help your consultations, they can also form part of your appraisal folder and might contribute towards the process of revalidation.

You may already have some idea about areas where you would like to start or consultation skills that would be useful to you and, if so, this section makes practical suggestions about how to go about this. If you are not yet sure where to start, Chapter 15 will help you to think about this, identifying learning needs and helping you to find somewhere to start. Subsequent chapters explore how and why some people learn differently from others and suggest different learning activities that might suit different people. Different methods of analysing consultations are explored and ways to give and receive feedback are discussed. The use of role play and video as tools to help with consultation analysis is also explored in some detail. The final chapter in this section will help you to put together a personal learning plan.

The tools and techniques suggested in this section are all tried and tested, and based on sound educational theory. The focus, however, is very much on a practical approach and on tools and techniques that can be used by any clinician, irrespective of the sort of practice in which they work. Those who wish to read and understand more about the educational theory behind the techniques may wish to use the references at the end of each chapter.

Chapter 15

Knowing where to start and what to learn

Alice came to a fork in the road. 'Which road do I take?' she asked. 'Where do you want to go?' responded the Cheshire cat. 'I don't know', Alice answered. 'Then', said the cat, 'It doesn't matter.'

Alice's Adventures in Wonderland, Lewis Carroll

'Excuse me, could you tell me how to get to Dublin, please?'
'Well ... if I were you, I wouldn't start from here.'

(Apocryphal Irish joke)

Key points

- The best place to start is the place you are at right now!
- Thinking about and reflecting on recent or memorable consultations will help you to identify areas of learning.
- The reflection can take several different forms and may be either alone or with a colleague.
- A personal learning log will help you to capture day-to-day learning points before they are lost.
- Knowing your preferred learning style will help you to think about the most effective way for you to learn.

So how do you know which skills or tools will be useful to add to your repertoire? A good place to start is by working out which sorts of consultation tend to cause you stress and difficulty. Just take a moment to think about three consultations you have had in the last few months or so that have been sub-optimal or stressful. You could jot down notes about what happened in each of them. Think about:

- the patient(s)
- yourself consulting that day
- the circumstances.

Use the following chart (which can be photocopied from Appendix 2) to help you identify what was memorable or difficult. Remember the feelings that you had at the time. Write these down too.

Patient	Yourself consulting that day	What happened?	How did you feel?	Any other observations or comments

Are there any patterns that start to emerge? You could keep a log like this for a week or a month, noting down significant consultations and look for themes. Does this give you pointers for identifying gaps in your skills or areas that it would be useful to work with? What new skills would be helpful to deal with such consultations in the future?

Keeping a learning log or journal

Some health professionals routinely use a learning log to reflect on what they are doing and to help flag up learning areas. The log can take several different physical forms, for example a notebook, Word document, PDA, tape recorder or any other storage device according to one's personal style or preference. Whatever you use, the idea is to note down, at the earliest possible opportunity, areas that you might want to think about and reflect on later. These might be:

- gaps that you identify in your clinical knowledge such as the latest guidelines in a particular clinical area
- skills that would be useful that you don't have now
- difficulties that arise in the process of the consultation.

These are sometimes referred to as PUNs and DENs (**P**atients' **U**nmet **N**eeds which flag up **D**octors' **E**ducational **N**eeds), originally described by Richard Eve (2003), a GP in Taunton. Ideally, you should make a note of these as soon as you identify them (in other words, during the consultation or between patients). If this is not realistic or feasible, perhaps because you are running late or have had a series of difficult consultations, then the next best time is immediately after surgery has finished – and by the end of the day at the latest. If you leave it any later than this you are likely to forget!

As well as noting and recording what happens in consultations, you could also make notes from other learning experiences:

- educational meetings that you attend
- written material from journals or books
- electronic learning, for example from the *BMJ*'s e-learning resource
- discussions with health colleagues in the practice, for example about problem patients, yours or theirs
- material that is highly relevant though not labelled or packaged as 'medical education', for example your thoughts and feelings after watching a television programme, going to the cinema, a concert or opera, or even visiting an art gallery. So many areas of the arts are loosely, or even directly, related to work in primary care and give interesting and illuminating insights.

At least once a fortnight, go through the list and work out how you will address particular areas. Again, look for common themes.

Possible action points

- If you don't keep a learning log or diary at the moment, try keeping one for a week.

- Experiment with different ways of recording your thoughts and feelings about the content and process of consultations, for example:
  - paper-based
  - computer programme such as a spreadsheet
  - voice recording on i-POD, cassette recorder, etc.
- Which method seems to suit you best?
- At the end of each surgery for a week, make notes about problem or difficult consultations.
- Schedule a time to review your diary, for example at the end of the week and perhaps with a colleague. What learning needs does it flag up? Think about ways that you might be able to meet these.

References and further reading

- Eve R. *PUNS and DENS – discovering learning needs in general practice*. Oxford: Radcliffe Medical Press; 2003.
- Grant J. Learning needs assessment: assessing the need. *BMJ*. 2002; **324**: 156–9.
- Powley E, Higson R. *The Arts in Medical Education – a practical guide*. Oxford: Radcliffe Publishing; 2005.
- www.john-lord.net/gp/dwt/index.htm (accessed 3 September 2005).

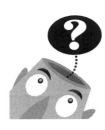

Chapter 16

How adults learn

Education is an admirable thing, but it is well to remember from time to time that nothing that is worth knowing can be taught.

The Critic as Artist, Oscar Wilde

Key points

- Adults learn in a different way from children.
- Adults learn best when their learning is related to a clearly perceived need and is based on their previous experience.
- Learning is usually an iterative process based on experience, reflection, making sense of what's happened and trying out new techniques.

Once you have an idea about what areas you might usefully tackle, how will you go about learning? Do you know how you learn best? Which is your favourite learning method? For example, different people prefer to:

- read a book or look up a journal article
- attend lectures or courses
- do a web-based module from an e-learning site
- talk to colleagues or partners about what they would do
- discuss the situation with a mentor or senior colleague
- simply reflect quietly and try and work out new strategies
- write guidelines or a patient information leaflet
- teach colleagues, GP registrars or members of the practice team.

Many educationalists believe that adults learn differently from children, though there is a view that it is simply that they are taught differently. Different people do, of course, learn in different ways and this will be explored later in this chapter. David Kolb (1984) produced a very useful descriptive cycle that is widely accepted as a good illustration of how adults learn. A common pattern is like this.

Practical experience

'This consultation with Mrs Horrible is going really badly. She's pressing my buttons and I'm just responding like an idiot. I don't know what it is about her that's getting my back up so badly. I just need to get her out of the room safely.'

Reflecting on what's happened

'This can't go on – I'm going to meet patients like her for the rest of my career. I need to find some strategies so that I can work with patients I don't like much whilst still being professional and helpful. I could do with some better ways of de-stressing too.'

Thinking what this means and how to do it better next time

> 'I need to learn some new skills here. Maybe this means I should go on a course, if there is one. In the meantime, I could debrief this with a colleague and perhaps rehearse some skills to try out another time. In terms of feeling better now – I'm going to walk round the block and get a cup of coffee.'

Trying it out again

- 'OK. Mrs Horrible is coming to see me again next week. This time I'll be more prepared for the encounter. I know which buttons she pressed last time, so I can be on the alert for these. I've worked out as well that one of the aspects of her that I reacted badly to was the resemblance she has to that ghastly teacher at school.'
- 'Hello, Mrs Horrible – nice to see you again. Come and sit down.'

This is then a cyclical activity because the clinician in the above is likely to reflect again after this consultation. The overall learning cycle looks like Figure 16.1 and different individuals will enter the cycle at different points.

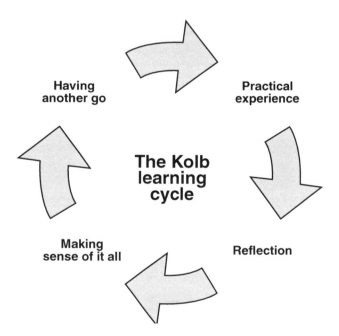

Figure 16.1 The Kolb learning cycle

Routes into the cycle

Practical experience

This might be the way into the learning cycle if you have had:

- a consultation that has gone badly

- interactions in other parts of your life that have gone well or badly, for example being on the receiving end of a good or bad medical consultation. Again, learning for consultations can come from other areas of your life such as a dysfunctional conversation with the garage mechanic or boiler engineer.

Reflection

On the other hand, you might find that a period of reflection gets you thinking about learning, for example:

- thinking about what has happened during your day
- a conversation over coffee with partners or colleagues
- writing in a journal or learning log.

Making sense of it all, or abstract conceptualisation

Sometimes there can be triggers to learning from other places such as:

- reading a book or watching a TV programme, film or play that gives you insight into patterns of how you behave
- a journal article that suggests a new approach to tackling difficult consultations.

Having another go, or active experimentation

Or you might just want to try out new or different consultation skills, such as:

- dealing with angry patients differently
- summarising back to every patient you see that morning
- practising the skill of getting patients to repeat back to you what they have understood about the management plan that you have agreed with them, without you sounding patronising
- imagining there's a video camera running in your consulting room and that you have to create a 'master' tape from this morning's surgery only – and if you're not successful, you'll be out of a job!

Different types of learner

So, all of us learn in a variety of different ways and, whilst no one is stuck in a box with a label on it, each of us will have a different preferred learning style. This is like knowing that you prefer to write with your right or left hand and that, whilst you could write with your non-dominant hand if you had to do so, it is generally much more straightforward and less taxing to write with your dominant hand.

This variation in learning styles helps to explain (at least in part) why some people may regard a particular learning event as wonderful and others will learn little from it. For example, activists may well get bored by lectures and theorists will hate being thrown in at the deep end or invited to role play. Knowing which style suits you best will help you to be able to choose learning activities that will be most effective for you. The four styles are commonly called activist, pragmatist, reflector and theorist. Each of these styles has a corresponding place in the Kolb learning cycle (*see* Figure 16.2).

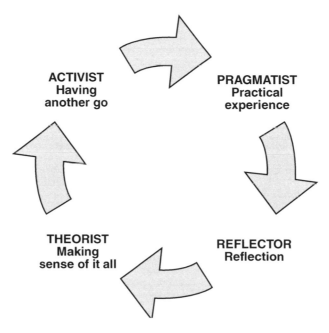

Figure 16.2 The four learning styles

Many primary care health professionals are activists and pragmatists with a smaller number who are reflectors and even fewer who are theorists. Honey and Mumford (1982) describe the characteristics of the four learning styles.

Activist

Activists are people who involve themselves fully in new experiences, enjoying the 'here and now'. They often relish change and thrive on challenge but can run out of steam with implementation.

Good learning activities for activists will have lots of variety and the chance to be involved in new experiences. Activists will tend to learn least from lectures and other passive experiences.

Pragmatist

Pragmatists are keen to try out ideas to see if they work in practice. They like to get on with things and act quickly and confidently. The most significant part of any learning for a pragmatist is the answer to the question, 'Does it work?'

Good learning activities for pragmatists are ones where there is a clear link between the educational material and the job, and there are obvious advantages such as saving time to the new techniques. Pragmatists learn least well from education that is 'all theory and no practice'.

Reflector

Reflectors like to stand back and think about their experiences before reaching conclusions. They often appear calm and unflappable and sometimes adopt a low profile, being quiet until they are sure what is going on.

Good learning activities for reflectors include the chance to observe others at work, down-time to review what has happened and think about what they have learnt, and activities that don't have tight deadlines. Reflectors learn least well when they are thrown in at the deep end, rushed or have little time to prepare.

Theorist

Theorists tend to think through problems logically. They prefer certainty to creativity and are uncomfortable with lateral thinking, subjectivity or anything trivial.

Good learning activities for theorists include structured situations with a clear purpose, the chance to question and probe ideas, and interesting ideas or concepts even though the relevance of these is not immediately apparent. Theorists learn least well when the activity is unstructured or the instructions are poor.

Example

A few years ago, when I was working as Course Organiser for the Leeds Vocational Training Scheme, a colleague and I ran an educational activity to help the registrars to discover their own learning styles. We first asked each of them to do the Honey and Mumford questionnaire to find out their preferred style and then divided them up into the four groups of activists, pragmatists, etc. We then gave each group a task – it's something of a party trick, which you may already know; but if you don't, you might want to have a go. The task is this:

> Take a sheet of A4 paper and make a hole in it large enough
> to pass over your head and body, so that you can step through
> the hole. You are not allowed to use scissors, sellotape, glue,
> paperclips or any other similar items.

We gave each group a pile of A4 paper and left them to it. The results were striking and illustrated to everyone the differences between the various styles.

The activists finished first. Within the first few seconds they were all noisily ripping paper and discarding sheets as it was clear that it wasn't working. They were using a trial and error approach and used far more paper than everyone else.

The pragmatists finished next. They had found a solution, but the hole was only in half the paper. It was then big enough to pass over the head of the smallest person in the group, so why bother making it any bigger?

The reflectors finished third. They had spent a long time talking and thinking about what to do before they ripped any paper. In the end they used only two sheets of paper – a 'dry run' and the real thing.

The theorists were unable to complete the task. They had used their time to discuss how they might do it but hadn't actually started to tackle it. They had also been trying to find cunning solutions that would fulfil the words of the instructions rather than the task, for example what was the nature of a 'hole' exactly?

This exercise illustrated beautifully the needs and strengths of different types of learners and helped them to work effectively in mixed groups for the rest of the six months, playing to each others' strengths and supporting each others' weaknesses.

(The solution is at the end of this chapter!)

Does it matter?

Having some idea about your preferred style of learning will help you to choose learning activities that suit you best. After all, if you enjoy what you learn and the way that you learn it, the learning is more likely to stay with you and be of use in the future.

If you want to learn more about learning styles and preferences, there are plenty of written and web-based materials to help you do this and these are referenced at the end of this chapter.

Possible action points

- Think about *anything* new that you have learnt during the last 12 months. This should not be confined to work-related activities. You could choose:
  - new hobbies or activities that you have taken up
  - learning about people around you and within relationships, including family and friends
  - learning about life and the world.
- Try and identify *how* you learnt. Was it through practical experience, reflecting afterwards, making sense of it or trying out something new?
- If you don't know what sort of learner you are, get a copy of the Honey and Mumford *Manual of Learning Styles* (1982) and find out.
- In the practice team or any other learning group that you are part of think about trying the hole-in-the-paper exercise. Remember to check first whether anyone has done this before and already knows the solution, and ask them to take a role as 'observer of the process'.

Solution to the 'hole in the paper' exercise

1. Take a sheet of A4 paper and fold it in half, long edge to long edge.
2. Make a series of tears starting at the folded edge and going nearly all the way across the paper.

3. Now make a series of tears starting at the opposite edge and running in between the first set of tears.
4. Now open out the sheet of paper and tear across the small joining sections, along the fold, to give a single large loop of paper. Easy when you know how!

References and further reading

- Honey P, Mumford A. *Manual of Learning Styles.* London: P Honey; 1982.
- Kolb DA. *Experiential Learning: experience as the source of learning and development.* Englewood Cliffs, NJ: Prentice Hall; Mentkowski M & Associates; 1984.
- Pietroni R. *The Toolbox for Portfolio Development – a practical guide for the primary care team.* Oxford: Radcliffe Medical Press; 2001.

Chapter 17

Working with colleagues to improve your consultation skills

I keep six honest serving-men
(They taught me all I knew);
Their names are What and Why and When
And How and Where and Who.

'The Elephant's Child', Rudyard Kipling

Key points

- Working with colleagues can be a very effective way of improving your consultation skills as they will have a slightly different perspective from you and can help to point out any blind spots that you may have.
- 'Colleagues' can be a single individual or a small group, and can be someone from a different healthcare profession, for example a practice nurse and a doctor working together.
- It is worth making agreements about how and when you will work together and setting some basic ground rules before you start.

Why work with colleagues?

Of course, you can work on your consultation skills alone, perhaps by reading this book or others on the consultation and trying out some of the suggestions, but working with colleagues offers additional opportunities.

- You will almost certainly discover that your colleague(s) consult(s) in a slightly different way from you. This will enable you to consider other ways of tackling consultations or parts of the consultation and may also mean that some of the ways you do things now are challenged.
- You will have the opportunity both to disclose to someone else (in other words, to tell them about aspects of your consultation skills that they don't know at the moment) and also to receive feedback from them.
- Feedback and disclosure are two very powerful tools for helping you to uncover blind spots in consultations skills – the areas that you don't know you don't know.

What you can do

There are many different ways that you can work with a colleague to improve your, and probably their, consultation skills. Here are some possible methods.

- **Videoing** Record a surgery and then look at the video tape together later. Remember you will need to get the patient's consent for this.
- **Audiotaping** This may be easier to arrange than videotaping, and also requires consent from the patient.
- **Random case analysis** Use the notes or computer records, picking cases at random and discussing aspects of the consultation skills.
- **Problem case analysis** Select cases that were particularly challenging and discuss them with a colleague.
- **Role play and skills rehearsal** Try out new skills or consultation techniques with a colleague in a safe learning environment, so that you are not using them live for the first time in an actual consultation.

A note on feedback and disclosure

Why are feedback and disclosure so significant in learning? You may have come across the Johari window, which is a pictorial representation of the fact that there are some things that we know about ourselves that others also know and some that others don't know. Equally there are some things that others know about us and we are aware of some of these but not others. *See* Figure 17.1.

	Known to self	**Not known to self**
Known to others	Arena – known to self and others	Blindspots – known to others but not to self
Not known to others	Façade – known to self but not known to others	Unknown to either self or others

Figure 17.1 Johari window

Feedback from others will reduce blind spots. Disclosing to others will reduce the area of the façade. Doing both will increase the area of the 'arena' and decrease the area of the unknown.

When to do it – finding the time

'I don't have the time' is an easy and justifiable excuse. All of us are increasingly busy and it can be difficult to set aside time to learn. But finding and protecting time to improve consultation skills is time well spent. It may well improve your efficiency in consultations as well as your (and the patients') satisfaction with them. A two-hour learning meeting with a colleague(s) once a month would be a good starting point.

Where?

So where will you work? This will be dictated by practical considerations and needs to be somewhere that is:

- accessible to you and others
- convenient and not too far to travel
- comfortable
- has video playback facilities, if you intend to use this as a medium for learning
- private, i.e. somewhere that you can work together without too much in the way of interruptions, and preferably none. If you work in your consulting room, put a 'Do not disturb' sign on the door.

How to go about it

Discussing your consultations with colleagues may feel threatening to a greater or lesser degree and there is no doubt that many doctors and nurses feel quite vulnerable about showing their consultation videos to others. For these reasons, it is important to develop some ground rules for this sort of educational activity and you should negotiate these with the person or people you intend to work with before you start. Clearly, the rules will vary according to the needs of the individuals but, typically, might include some or all of the following.

Confidentiality

- **Of patient material**, obviously.
- **'What's said in this room, stays in this room'** In other words an agreement that neither of you is going to spill the beans to others about your weaknesses, vulnerabilities or problems in the practice or with colleagues. It may well also be worth agreeing what material can be taken out of the room, perhaps to add it to your portfolio of learning or personal learning plan, or as material for discussion at your appraisal.
- **Limits of confidentiality** As with any encounter between two health professionals (or any other human beings, with the exception of Catholic priests), confidentiality is not absolute. If you discover during the consultation that your colleague is doing something actively dangerous or breaching ethics, you have a responsibility to do something about it and, in the worst possible case (or if someone completely refuses or is unable to change unacceptable behaviour), this could ultimately extend to you talking to the local Clinical Governance lead or even the GMC. This, I know, sounds very scary but it is a worst-possible-case scenario, which happens very, very rarely. Bringing problems into the open does, at least, mean that people can become more aware of any areas of difficulty so that they have the opportunity to learn and change. It is, however, worth discussing early, well before there is a difficult situation, so that you are both clear about this.

Feedback

- Agreement about giving and receiving feedback safely.
- Methods of feedback that will be used.

Ways of giving and receiving feedback will be covered in detail in Chapter 20.

Time

- How often will you meet?
- How will the time be shared?
- Protection of the time, i.e. avoiding times when either one of you is on call.

Valuing difference

There is no single right way to consult and very few absolutes. The fact that I deal with a situation this way and you deal with it differently (and the patients are equally safe and happy) does not mean that I am right and you are wrong. The differences are interesting and something to be valued rather than criticised.

Who to work with

Who will you choose to work with to improve your consultation skills? Whoever it is, it is likely that there will be some core conditions that must be met if you are to be able to work together effectively.

- **Availability** You need to find someone who has or is willing to find or create regular time to work with you. This means that it is likely that they will be geographically close to you and perhaps already working in your practice or in a neighbouring practice.
- **Willingness** As well as being available, they need to have the willingness and enthusiasm to work with you.
- **Like-mindedness** When undertaking this sort of work, it is useful to have a colleague whom you respect and with whom you see eye to eye.
- **Interest in consultations** Clearly, if the person you choose to work with is not all that interested in the consultation, it is unlikely that the working relationship will be sustained very long.
- **Trust** You are going to be working together in some potentially sensitive areas, so it is important that you choose someone you trust.

This sort of helping relationship tends to work best when there is an equality of learning. There will be times during the process of learning when you may have the relationship of teacher and learner, but so long as these roles are reversed and reciprocated, so that both parties have an equal turn in each role, there will be equality. An unequal relationship is less likely to be sustainable. The situation where one party is always the learner and the other is always the teacher can work for a specific, defined (usually paid) contract, for example the GP registrar and trainer for six months. However, it is much less useful for adult learning because it will get overlaid with feelings of gratitude, duty, guilt or just increasing boredom, and these feelings will tend to contaminate the learning and make it unsustainable.

Some suggestions about who to work with

- **A colleague in the practice** This might be someone in your own professional group but could well be a different health professional, for example a nurse and doctor working together.
- **A group of colleagues in the practice** You could set aside an 'educational hour' each week when several colleagues get together to review their consultations. This might be a group of doctors, nurses, a mixed clinical team, GP registrars or others.
- **The whole clinical team** This can work really well in terms of involving everyone – nurses, doctors and any other health professionals – but can also mean that the work is done on a more superficial level. Sometimes nurses, in particular, can find it intimidating to show their consultation videos in front of doctors. Experience on the 'Naked Consultation' course has demonstrated that nurses and doctors tend to have very similar skills and there is certainly no need for anxiety!
- **A colleague in a neighbouring practice** This can have the advantage that their working conditions and patient group may well be different from yours.
- **A young principals' group.**
- **A group of nurses** from neighbouring practices.
- **Former colleagues** from your VTS or people you work with in the out-of-hours' service or at an outpatient clinic.
- **Other members of a nurse practitioner group.**

Chapter 18 outlines how you might go about discussing cases with colleagues. Following this, there is guidance on feedback, then role play and ways that you might use video.

Possible action points

- Think about who you could work with.
- Could you set up a learning group in the practice? Are there like-minded colleagues who you could discuss this with?
- Set a realistic timescale for getting started with this.

Further reading

- Luft J, Ingham H. *The Johari Window: a graphic model of interpersonal awareness.* Proceedings of the Western Training Laboratory in Group Development. Los Angeles: UCLA; 1955.

Case discussion

Key points

- Discussion of problem cases with colleagues can be very useful, and happens sporadically in many practices.
- Discussion of cases picked at random, that didn't cause you problems, can be even more useful and can help to unearth blind spots – the areas that we don't know we don't know.

Methods of analysing consultations

Two common tried and tested methods frequently used by trainers and registrars when teaching and learning about the consultation are problem case analysis and random case analysis. These are both good methods and work well for peer learning on a one-to-one basis as well as for groups of health professionals, for example a practice clinical team.

Problem case analysis

Problem case analysis is an extension of what goes on in many practices over coffee, lunch or clinical meetings.

- 'I had a really difficult consultation this morning – felt absolutely drained afterwards.'
- 'I'm stuck here – this patient has symptoms that just don't seem to fit together and yet I'm sure there's something wrong.'
- 'I'm sure I should know the latest guidelines on hypertension, but this patient is already on three drugs and I'm just not sure what to do next. Any thoughts?'
- 'I ran *really* late this morning ...'
- 'I heard some really shocking news this morning.'

This unscheduled, ad hoc debriefing and sharing of problem cases is extremely useful and certainly one of the reasons why I work in a group practice and would never wish to be single-handed. It has the advantages of:

- immediacy – problems can be tackled the same day or within hours or minutes whilst they are still fresh
- an opportunity to offload any negative feelings of anger, frustration or sadness so that they don't accumulate and lead to burnout or worse
- helping to cement relationships within the practice team. Today it might be me offloading and asking for help, but tomorrow it may be my partner or colleague who is doing the same. There is mutual trust and support and these are valuable.

The main disadvantage is that colleagues may not have the time to listen. On a busy day, there may be other pressing calls on one's time such as extra patients, visits, hospital clinics to go to, etc.

Scheduled time for learning, focused on problem cases, will mean that there is protected time to discuss them. Although it may be less immediate than ad-hoc debriefing, sometimes the fact that the cases are discussed a few days later than they happened can mean that the health professional involved has already had new insights or thoughts about what happened – what is lost through lack of immediacy may be repaid by reflection.

Random case analysis

Random case analysis can sometimes be even more interesting than problem case analysis. It means that cases that would normally be glossed over as 'too easy/too boring/over in 2 minutes/just a repeat prescription' are discussed. This can lead to surprising enlightenments in areas such as attitudes and is a very useful route to locate blind spots.

What are random cases?

Random cases are, by definition, selected entirely randomly. This means that they are not chosen for discussion because they are:

- interesting
- 'difficult'
- challenging
- show off your amazing diagnostic skills
- a patient you know well
- or any one of a hundred other 'non-random' reasons.

How do you select cases randomly?

It should be quite straightforward to choose cases at random but watching videos of trainers and registrars undertaking this sort of case analysis, it is apparent that many of the cases discussed are not random at all! For example:

- 'Let's look at your list of patients this morning. Ah yes, I see you had Mr Brown. He's one of my regulars. Tell me what he came in with today!'
- 'Let's look at the notes of patients you saw this morning. Ah yes, the first, second and third all seem to have had interesting problems. Let's talk about them.'
- 'We said we'd do a random case analysis today. Which patients would you like to talk about?'

Better ways of selecting random cases are:

- write the numbers 1–20 (or whatever) on separate pieces of paper and draw some 'out of the hat'. You then discuss the patients who came in third, ninth and twelfth (or whatever)
- use a random number generator website on the computer, for example random.org.

Choosing a theme for the discussion

It can be helpful to select a theme on which to base your discussions.

- **'Beginnings' in consultations** What happened? Gambit or curtain raiser? How long was the patient allowed to talk for? Had they said all they needed to at this point?
- **Cues given by the patient** Notice if, when and how these were picked up by the consulting health professional.
- **Getting information from patients** What skills were used?
- **Patients' health beliefs** What were they and how do you know this?
- **Summarising back** Did you do it? If so, how? Did the patient fully agree with your summary, in other words did everything about their verbal and non-verbal behaviour say an unequivocal 'yes'? If not, what did you do?
- **Giving information to patients** What language did you use? Did you use their own vocabulary of nouns and verbs? Did you take into account the way that they see, hear and/or feel the world?
- **Checking understanding** Did you check understanding about the diagnosis and the management plan?
- **Safety-netting** Did you use a three-point safety net?
- **Uncertainty** How did you manage it? Think about your own uncertainties as well as the patient's.
- **Endings.**
- **Recording notes** Looking now at the consultation, what was recorded? Was it Read coded? If it was a significant problem, was it recorded in the patient's summary?

How many random cases to cover

In an hour's discussion, three or four cases are about right. This allows about 10 minutes to discuss each case, either from the notes or by watching a consultation video, and then 10 further minutes for discussion. Trying to cover more cases than this can mean that any discussion is too brief to be effective.

Whose cases – yours or mine?

If two of you are working together, you could either alternate sessions so that one week you look at one person's consultations and the next week at the other person's, or you could alternate the consultations that you look at during a particular session. Juxtaposing two people's consultations like this can be a very effective way of flagging up and highlighting similarities and differences, and therefore learning points, from each others' consultations.

Extrapolation – the 'what ifs'

One of the really useful aspects of random case analysis is that it allows you to extrapolate from the patient you are discussing and consider other possibilities. You are limited only by your imagination!

Example

A video has been watched of a patient who had requested antibiotics for a sore throat over the phone and had been told to make an appointment to be seen (which he was reluctant to do, being a busy person). In the consultation, he is initially angry but later settles down and leaves with advice and a deferred prescription. Some of the 'what ifs' covered in the discussion might be what if he had:

- become even more angry and the doctor or nurse had felt physically threatened during the consultation
- been unwilling to accept a 'deferred' prescription
- had six similar episodes of 'sore throat' in the last year
- been asking for diazepam in the same demanding way
- disclosed that the sore throat was a cover for telling you about an unpleasant penile discharge he had had ever since an 'encounter' in Bangkok and this was the real reason that he wanted antibiotics.

Ending the session

At the end of the time reviewing random cases, it is a good idea to allow 5–10 minutes for summarising what has gone on, reflecting on what has been learnt and flagging up any learning needs that have been identified but that weren't fully addressed in the session.

Possible action points

- Plan to discuss cases picked at random, as well as those where there have been difficulties.
- Choose a theme to help to focus your discussions.
- Be realistic in the numbers of cases that you choose to discuss – three or four in an hour is enough.

Further reading

- McEvoy P. *Educating the Future GP – the course organisers' handbook*. Oxford: Radcliffe Medical Press; 1998.
- Middleton P, Field S. *The GP Training Handbook*. Oxford: Radcliffe Medical Press; 2000.
- www.gp-training.net/training/theory/rca2.htm (accessed 1 May 2006).
- www.trainer.org.uk/members/tools/case_analysis.htm (accessed 1 May 2006).

Chapter 19

Getting and giving effective feedback

Key points

- Used effectively, feedback can be a very powerful learning tool.
- It is well worth learning both how to give and how to receive effective feedback.
- There are different methods of giving feedback, and some of these are described here.

Introduction

So would you like some feedback? In fact, can I give you some feedback, if it's all the same to you? Well, quite clearly I can't because I don't know you and can't assess your performance, comment on your behaviour, praise or criticise you. But how do you respond or feel about being asked this sort of question? How do you feel about feedback in general?

'Feedback' is a word that sometimes has negative feelings attached to it. From time to time it is used as a weasel word to dress up criticism and as an excuse to legitimise verbally aggressive, humiliating or even bullying behaviour. 'Do you mind if I give you some feedback?' can mean:

- 'Actually I don't really care whether you mind or you don't, I'm going to tell you anyway. I've asked you the question, but it's rhetorical – it does not need an answer (whether 'yes' or 'no') and I'm going to tell you just what I think about you.'
- 'I am about to tell you off.'
- 'I am really quite angry and you are about to be on the receiving end of my sharp tongue.'

Used well, effectively and in a safe way, feedback can give us real insights into other people's views of our behaviour, in a way that can help us to change and develop. Good feedback includes both positive statements – identifying what we have done well – and also flags up areas that have had a more negative impact and could be a focus for change.

There are different methods of giving people feedback and, if you are working with a colleague on your consultation skills, it would be a very good idea to agree the methods and the rules first. There are some rules of feedback that are non-negotiable, for example:

- **Feedback should be about behaviour not about the person or their personality.** 'I noticed when you interrupted Mrs Brown she looked rather downcast and seemed a bit quiet after that' is acceptable – the behaviour (interruption) is highlighted. 'You are incredibly dominating and overbearing – no wonder all the patients complain about you' is unacceptable – it makes a comment about the health professional's personality as well as being an unacceptable and almost certainly incorrect generalisation.

- **Feedback should be as close in time to the event as possible.** 'I saw Mr Smith myself today and he told me, in no uncertain terms, that you upset him in a consultation you had last year.' This is not very helpful because I can't now remember Mr Smith, let alone the consultation when I am supposed to have upset him, so I just feel criticised without being able to respond or even defend my actions. This is unacceptable. On the other hand, if you tell me about something that a patient told you happened in a consultation this morning, I'm much more likely to be able to understand and make sense of the feedback. This feedback is acceptable.
- **Feedback should describe what the observer saw, heard or felt, rather than being judgemental.** 'When Ms Jones was telling you how upset she is about her marriage and started to look tearful, I noticed that you seemed uncomfortable and changed the subject straight away' is acceptable. 'Are you always so insensitive?' is not.
- **Feedback should take place in privacy**, not in front of a load of observers who are not really involved at all, otherwise it can be very threatening and make the receiver defensive rather than receptive.
- **Feedback should include checks of clarity and understanding** as in a consultation, otherwise you have no way of knowing whether what was heard matches what you think you said.
- **Feedback should be invited and welcomed, not imposed.** Does the person in front of you actually want feedback? Ask them first! Unwelcome and unsolicited feedback may occasionally be necessary but is likely only to relieve the feelings, frustration or anger of the giver, rather than being something that the receiver can use in order to help them change.

Models for giving feedback

Sandwich model

This model sandwiches negative or critical feedback between two layers of praise.

1. This is what you did well.
2. This is what I think went less well or could be done differently.
3. This is how it might be achieved, given your strengths and positive behaviours.

The advantages of this model are that it is easy to remember the structure and the unconscious brain is less defensive and more receptive if it is praised first and last. The disadvantages are that it is simplistic and doesn't really involve the learner in the feedback.

Club sandwich model (multilayers)

This offers a more dynamic, interactive approach to feedback.

1. What do you think you did well?
2. This is what I saw you do well.
3. Is there anything that you might do differently in the future?

4. This is what I think you might do differently.
5. Do you have any thoughts about how you might go about doing things differently?
6. Here are some suggestions about how I think you might go about doing things differently.
7. What do you think you might try first?

The advantages are that the learner is involved as an equal participant and clear ways forward for the learner to change are identified. The disadvantages are that sometimes people ignore or blot out everything before step 4 – 'Cut the waffle and get to the "but"!'

SET-GO model

1. What did you, the learner **see**?
2. What **else** did I, the trainer see?
3. What do you, the learner **think** about this?
4. What **goals** can we now set?
5. What **offers** have we got to achieve these goals?

This model gets straight to the points raised by the learner and focuses on solutions. However, it can be easy to forget the positive and focus only on the negative.

Receiving feedback

So far we have concentrated on giving feedback but there are behaviours and skills that help you to receive feedback in a positive and helpful way.

- Agree the rules first.
- Make sure the time, place and setting are right.
- Work with someone whose opinion you respect.
- You have to want it! If you really don't want feedback, then say so. Unsolicited feedback can be unwelcome and even damaging.
- Think about whether you agree with what is said, or not. If you don't, you should state this and check out your own opinion with the giver of the feedback.
- Be receptive. What can you learn from this feedback about how your behaviour is perceived by others?

Other forms of feedback

Sometimes, of course, you receive direct feedback from patients, which you may or may not have asked for and which may be verbal or in writing, for example:

- verbal expressions of thanks from patients, often about previous consultations that have been significant for them or have helped them
- written or verbal complaints from patients
- written expressions of thanks such as letters or cards
- solicited feedback in writing, for example a patient satisfaction survey.

This feedback is often quite 'raw' in that most patients don't know the rules about feedback, but it is usually honest and is well worth reading, reflecting on and discussing with colleagues.

Possible action points

- Think about circumstances in which you give feedback to others. Are you happy with how you do it or could it be improved?
- Think about occasions when you have received feedback. Did it enable you to change? If so, what was helpful. If not, why not?
- Practise giving feedback in an educational setting such as a learning group. Ask for feedback about how you do it!

Further reading

- Kaprielian V, Gradison M. Effective use of feedback. *Family Medicine.* 1998; **30**(6): 406–7.
- Kurtz S, Silverman J, Draper J. *Teaching and Learning Communication Skills in Medicine.* Oxford: Radcliffe Medical Press; 1998. 2nd edn; 2004.
- LeBaron S, Jernick J. Evaluation as a dynamic process. *Family Medicine.* 2000; **32**(1): 13–14.
- Pendleton D, Schofield T, Tate P. *The Consultation: an approach to learning and teaching.* Oxford: Oxford University Press; 1984.
- Silverman J, Draper J, Kurtz S. The Calgary-Cambridge approach to communication skills teaching II: The SET-GO method of descriptive feedback. *Education for General Practice.* 1997; **8**: 16–23.
- Silverman J, Kurtz S, Draper J. *Skills for Communicating with Patients.* Oxford: Radcliffe Medical Press; 1998. 2nd edn; 2004.

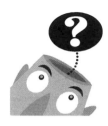

Chapter 20

Using role play to help with consultation techniques

Key points

- Role playing with a colleague can be an effective and useful way of working out what happened, and why, in a difficult consultation.
- Some people are anxious about using role play but used properly and effectively it can be a powerful tool for change.
- It is important to get out of role at the end of a role-play exercise. Remember to do this every time.

Introduction

Role play can be a very useful technique to help you explore difficulties that have occurred in consultations as well as rehearse or try out new skills in a safe environment. Some people, I know, have negative feelings associated with role play, particularly if they have had past experiences of being put on the spot, unable to say 'no' despite the fact that they really didn't want to be involved and have then been uncomfortable or even embarrassed when performing in front of others. It doesn't need to be like this! Role play between two individuals as part of a helping and learning relationship can be a powerful but safe tool.

Using role play to analyse difficult consultations

One of the most effective ways of starting to understand what has happened or even gone wrong in a complex consultation is to role play it with a colleague afterwards. If you were the healthcare practitioner in a particularly difficult consultation, then you could take the role of the patient in the same consultation, whilst someone else assumes the practitioner role. In becoming the patient, consider as many aspects as you can.

- How did the patient look when they came in?
- What was their speech like?
- What emotions do you think were going on?
- Was there a point when their behaviour changed?
- What do you know about their background and how might this impact on the way they present themselves in the consultation?

Clearly the consultation won't be an exact re-run of the difficult one you have just had, but it may well be even more effective as a learning tool through being slightly different. There are three possible reasons for this.

- In assuming the role of the difficult patient, you may start to gain insight into what made them so unhappy, angry or muddled up in the consultation.

- Your helper taking the practitioner role will almost certainly handle the consultation slightly differently from the way you did and this may well give you new ideas and thoughts about strategies that work, as well as those that don't.
- When you and your colleague debrief the consultation together afterwards, you will both have experienced being on the receiving end of the 'patient' so you will usefully be able to compare experiences. It is very likely that through doing this you will be able to come to a deeper understanding of what happened and why.

You can also try out different strategies:

- If the practitioner makes a different intervention at a particular point, how does this affect the outcome? How does the 'patient' respond to this?
- The 'patient' can also give feedback about how they feel at particular points and offer suggestions to the healthcare professional.

Using role play to practise new consultation techniques

Another use of role play is in practising new or different consultation techniques. It may be that, either through reading this book or through working with colleagues, you have been wondering about using different tools or techniques in your consultations. Some of these may be ones that are easy to practise in many or most consultations such as:

- opening the consultation in a different way
- summarising back to the patient
- finding out the patient's health beliefs
- checking that the patient has understood what you have said by getting them to repeat it back to you in their own words.

But there may be other skills where the opportunity for practice only comes around occasionally – and where you may be particularly keen for any technique that you use to *work* rather than lead you into difficulties or unknown places. This might apply to:

- breaking bad news
- managing a patient's anger
- dealing with a professional colleague who consults you about a difficult problem such as depression or addiction.

Role playing these situations, before they arise, would allow you to get skills practice and feedback within a safe environment. In this situation, you could take the role of health professional whilst your colleague acts the role of patient. You could then swap the roles around if you wish so that you each have the experience of both sides (or corners) of the desk.

Keeping it safe

As with any educational activity, it is important to set up a few rules and boundaries in advance. This will help to keep the role play safe and therefore make it more educationally effective. The rules don't need to be clever or complicated – just a straightforward agreement of some key issues such as:

- how long you are going to spend doing this (for example 10 minutes for a consultation, with an agreement that you will stop and check out at that point before deciding whether or not to continue)
- confidentiality, as usual, of patient material and of whatever happens in the room
- agreement about what sort of feedback you will give to each other.

De-roling

It is important to remember to come out of the role and back into yourself properly at the end of any session like this, particularly if emotions have been running high and you have really got yourself into the part! One effective way to do this is to state out loud who you are and three things about yourself that are quite different from the patient, for example:

> 'I'm Liz. Unlike Mrs Challenging, I'm not living on the poverty line; I don't have four children under the age of five and I really enjoy listening to live jazz.'

Possible action points

- Role play gets easier with practice – just do it!
- Next time you have a really difficult consultation, use the techniques described in this chapter to 'become' the patient temporarily and work with a colleague to discover how they would have handled the situation.

Further reading

- Atherton JS. *Learning and Teaching: Exercises: role play.* 2003. Available online www.dmu.ac.uk/~jamesa/teaching/exercises_roleplay.htm (accessed 24 April 2005).

Chapter 21

Videoing

Key points

- Videoing is one of the most useful of all tools for learning and teaching about the consultation.
- There are some rules that need to be adhered to: getting informed consent and permission from patients, and about how to look safely at each others' videos.

Introduction

When did you last video a surgery and look at it? Videoing is a tool that many health professionals use when they are learning about consultation skills, for example as GP registrars or as trainee nurse practitioners, but few use it after they have passed summative assessment, final exams or the equivalent process. This is a shame and a missed opportunity. Looking at videos of consultations, either alone or with others, is a very useful way of enhancing skills.

- You can watch your own skills and behaviour, and observe the whole range of techniques that you use.
- You can identify good areas and skills as well as those that might benefit from some attention.
- You will almost certainly find that you start to notice small or minimal cues that were made by the patient that weren't really apparent at the time of the consultation, for example the jokey or throwaway line that they came out with just as they sat down again after the examination and whilst you were turned away entering information on the computer. Noticing these escapees from the internal policemen on video is a good first step towards becoming more aware of them in the consultation.
- You can watch, pause, rewind, replay the video and notice how the patient responded to particular interventions that you made.
- You can be a fly on the wall and watch what was happening to the patient whilst you were turned away from them, perhaps getting the auriscope, entering data on the computer or even going out of the room. At times, this can be even more revealing than you might expect. A colleague of mine was videoing a surgery, went out of the room for a few minutes trying to find a letter/report and had the camera running the whole time. When he came to play the video, he was shocked to notice that the patient had started crying when he was absent and only stopped moments before he re-entered the room. He had not noticed this in the actual consultation at all.

The rules

There are some straightforward rules about videoing, in order to protect patients by ensuring that they have consented and that their privacy is respected.

- Patients need to be told when they book their appointment that the consultation will be videoed for educational purposes.
- When they check in at the desk, they should be given an information sheet telling them why they will be videoed, what will happen to the video (for example, who will see it) and asked to sign a consent form if they agree to this. Sample forms that you can photocopy and use are included in Appendix 2.
- At the end of the videoed consultation, the receptionist should check with the patient that they are still happy for the video to be used or whether they would now prefer it to be erased. This second consent mustn't be done by the clinician they consulted because some patients may feel obliged to say that the video can be kept when they would prefer it to be erased.
- Any examination that involves removing any clothing at all should not be videoed. If you can, keep the camera running but put the lens cap on it so that the picture is blank but the sound continues because, of course, the process of the consultation continues throughout this time.
- It goes without saying that any videos should be stored safely and securely and wiped clean once they are finished with.

How, when and where

If at all possible, arrange to video a surgery in your own consulting room. This will ensure that you are in as familiar an environment as possible and that the consultation skills you see will not be affected by lack of fluency due to a different location or inability to lay your hands on a piece of kit that you need. It's also more practical and easier than having to negotiate use of a different room – so you are more likely to do it!

If you are not familiar with the equipment, ask a friend or colleague to teach you how to use it. Position the camera so that it is as unobtrusive as possible but allows both you and the patient to be seen clearly in the frame. Before you start, borrow a receptionist or colleague for a few moments and exchange a few words whilst sitting in the two chairs – yours and the patient's. Playback the interaction and check again that both parties are in view and that the microphone is switched on and picking up sound effectively. This may sound obvious, but there is nothing worse than having captured a really interesting consultation on the video that you then find is switched off, out of battery, inaudible, too dark or one person is completely out of the frame. If sound quality is a problem, obtain and use a desktop microphone, or use a directional microphone on or near the camera.

If you haven't videoed for a while or are new to it, plan your early videos for surgeries where you are likely to be undisturbed and as unstressed as possible. For example, avoid choosing the day that you are on call or a surgery where you are always under pressure, perhaps because not many doctors are consulting then. As you get more comfortable with video, recording these more difficult surgeries may well be very enlightening. But for the moment, whilst you get comfortable with the process, stick to straightforward ones. There will still be plenty of material!

Altering consultation lengths when videoing

Should you lengthen your consultation booking intervals when videoing? Some doctors and nurses do this as a matter of routine, adding on 5 or 10 minutes to their normal interval. This may feel more comfortable and less rushed, but the disadvantage is that you will not be recording your normal time-pressured consultations. It's much easier to have a really good consultation in 20 minutes than in 10 minutes, but the idea of video is to help you to find ways to improve your ordinary consultations, not the special double-length ones. It may be reasonable to lengthen your consultation booking interval when you are first videoing, but try and cut this back down to your normal length as soon as you can.

Looking at videos

Looking at your own videos can be uncomfortable or even scary at first and you might want to look at the first ones alone and in private. Doing this and nothing else will almost certainly flag up areas of learning. If you want to learn more, you will need to involve a colleague in order to get feedback and to allow you to disclose – the two powerful tools that help to increase learning by taking you into blind spots and unknown areas. Inevitably, this means that someone else will need to watch your consultations with you as well! Every doctor and health professional that I have ever met has worried about this and the fear tends to be that the other person watching the video will think that you are a rubbish doctor or nurse and will say so and totally undermine your confidence! There need to be some agreed rules to provide a safe and effective environment and you might well like to start with the ones described here, which are called Pendleton's rules. For the purposes of clarity, I have called the person whose video is being watched 'the learner' and the person who is watching their videos with them 'the colleague'.

Pendleton's rules

1. Colleague and learner watch the video together in silence.
2. At the end of the particular consultation, any factual matters are clarified, for example what was written on the prescription, if this isn't obvious from the video.
3. The learner goes first with good points. This is crucial! Most people watching their own videos will seize on anything that they weren't happy with or that went less well. Focusing on good points first makes sure that you look for them and explicitly acknowledge them.
4. The colleague goes next with good points. Again, it is likely that the learner will have not consciously noted all of these and it is effective and helpful to have someone state them.
5. The learner then states any areas which, with hindsight, they think weren't so good or wish they had done differently.
6. Finally, the colleague makes suggestions or recommendations, not criticisms, about areas for possible change.

Problem-based interviewing

This is the name given to another very useful way of looking at consultations that focuses on finding out what the patient has *really* come about. It encourages the clinician to consider more than the patient's words and description of their problems, thinking as well about what they observed, heard and felt themselves during the consultation. In other words, the learner is helped and encouraged to use all the sources of information available to them. This method was first described by Art Lesser (1985) from McMaster University and adapted by David Goldberg and Linda Gask (1987) in Manchester for use in consultation skills teaching.

This method has the advantage of being more dynamic and active than the Pendleton model and it can offer space and scope for 'what ifs'. In focusing attention on the clinician's thoughts and feelings, it can help to raise awareness of the usefulness of these during the process of consultation.

1. The learner selects the consultation and identifies issues that they want to focus or concentrate on. The observing colleague might well need to tease these out a bit to produce a learning agenda.

Example

Learner: I'd like to look at the consultation with Mr B. It was difficult and I'd appreciate some help with it.
Colleague: Difficult? What made it difficult?
Learner: Well, I just didn't get anywhere, we seemed to be going round in circles.
Colleague: Circles?
Learner: Every time I suggested treatment options, he just went back to how awful the symptoms were.
Colleague: I wonder why that was. Did you find out what he was really worried about?
Learner: Well, I didn't think there was anything much wrong, but perhaps I should have concentrated more on what he was thinking.
Colleague: Well, perhaps that's a good place to start. We could look at the tape and see what cues he is giving out.

---

2. Both parties then watch the tape and either of them can stop it at any time.
3. Whilst watching the tape they should each focus on what actually happens on the tape, for example the patient's verbal and non-verbal behaviour and cues, and the clinician's response to these.
4. Although clinical content is clearly important, wherever possible you should focus on the consultation skills used.
5. The tape can be stopped at any time to:
   - draw attention to a skill which was demonstrated
   - suggest something which could have been done differently, but the person who stops the tape must offer an alternative form of words or behaviours. This is likely to be a dynamic and interactive process between the learner and their colleague in that there may be several

alternatives and formulating the best response may well be a collaborative process.

6. When the tape is stopped, it can be helpful to explore 'what ifs' and to think what would have happened differently if an alternative route had been taken at that point.

Possible action points

- One of the biggest challenges about videoing is simply getting started. Plan a date in the near future, practise with the equipment first, then just go ahead!
- Videoing gets easier with practice. You may feel inhibited or anxious at first but this will soon pass with practice.
- Remember the rules when giving feedback about someone else's videos.

References and further reading

- Gask L, McGrath G, Goldberg D, Millar T. Improving the psychiatric skills of established general practitioners: evaluation of group teaching. *Medical Education.* 1987; **21**: 362–3.
- Lesser A. Problem-based interviewing in general practice: a model. *Medical Education.* 1985; **19**(4): 299–304.
- www.abersychan.demon.co.uk/video.htm
- www.skillscascade.com/courses/one_to_one.htm

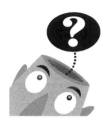

Chapter 22

Consultation skills and the RCGP

Most candidates know how to pass with merit because they tell the oral examiners that they consult in a patient-centred way. Most insist they explore their patient's beliefs, listen actively, seek out their agendas, discover about them as human beings, examine them properly, share their understanding, involve them in their own management and share decisions with them. The current problem is that 95% of candidates tell the oral examiners this is what they do but only 10% actually demonstrate this behaviour on the submitted videotape.

RCGP website

Key points

Not surprisingly, the Royal College of General Practitioners (RCGP) views effective consultation skills as very important and, at the time of writing, assessment of these forms a key part of both the MRCGP examination (which tends to be taken by GP registrars [GPRs] in training and those who have not long finished their training) and the Membership by Assessment of Performance (MAP). The latter is a more practical assessment of performance and is an alternative route to the MRCGP, more suitable for doctors who have been in practice for a while.

The current MRCGP consultation skills assessment will be phased out over the next few years but it is likely that there will continue to be some sort of video assessment of consultation skills, forming part of the proposed workplace-based assessment.

One common complaint by doctors in training is that they find it very difficult to produce a consultation video that lasts less than 15 minutes (the cut-off for the present exam) and yet still includes all the relevant criteria. I have also heard registrars talk about having to tick the boxes and jump through the hoops of the exam when, of course, real doctors don't consult like that at all. This is a shame – the exam tests many of the skills that can and should be part of any effective doctor's consultation toolkit and it is perfectly possible to use these in many (though not all) ordinary ten-minute consultations.

The framework

The framework for the assessment of consultation skills looks remarkably familiar, because it is a pared-down version of most consultation models.

- Discover the reason for the patient's attendance.
- Define the clinical problem(s).
- Explain the problem(s) to the patient.

- Address the patient's problem(s).
- Make effective use of the consultation.

Each element of the framework is broken down into several performance criteria and some of these are rated 'pass' (P) and others 'merit' (M). In order to pass, it is necessary to demonstrate each pass criterion four times in the total of seven consultations. At the time of writing, the following criteria are used.

Discover the reason for the patient's attendance

There are three parts to this, each one having a performance criterion that needs to be met.

Elicit an account of the symptoms

'The doctor is seen to encourage the patient's contribution at appropriate points in the consultation.' (P)

This is about demonstrating active listening skills:

- minimal encouragers
- use of silence
- reflecting back to the patient
- echoing
- facilitating the patient to 'go on'.

There is also a merit criterion here:

'The doctor is seen to respond to cues that lead to a deeper understanding of the problem.' (M)

Note there are two parts to this and it is not enough, for the exam, to notice and respond to the cues if that doesn't then lead to a deeper understanding of the problem! The sorts of cues that you might respond to are:

- a patient's non-verbal communication, such as:
  - 'I noticed that you looked really sad just then.'
  - 'You seem quite tense and anxious.'
- something that is apparent from the records, for example:

  'It's really quite a while since you've been to the surgery – a couple of years or so?'

- a connection that you have noticed but the patient might not have:

  'You've mentioned a couple of times now about your friend with cancer – is that, by any chance, something you might be worried about yourself?'

If an exploration like this leads to greater understanding of the patient's problems, then the merit criterion is met.

Obtain relevant items of social and occupational circumstances

'The doctor uses appropriate psychological and social information to place the complaint(s) in context.' (P)

In other words, you think about how the patient's occupation, home life, relationships and emotional well-being affect and are affected by their problem and ask an appropriate question:

- 'You're a teacher, I think. Are you missing much time off work with the headaches? Is that causing problems at school?'
- 'You've been very stressed and anxious, and I know you've already told me about some of the things at work that contribute to that. Are there any problems at home as well?'
- 'This bad back of yours has been troublesome for a while. I was just wondering how being off work for so long is making you feel?'

Explore the patient's health understanding

> 'The doctor explores the patient's health understanding.' (P)

This is about finding out the patient's health belief system, which is much easier once you've started to practise asking every patient what they think might be wrong with them. For example:

- 'You've had this tummy pain for a few weeks now. I was just wondering whether you've had any thoughts or worries yourself about what might be wrong?'
- 'Can I just check with you – when you booked the appointment to see me today, what was going through your mind about what might be wrong or how I might be able to help?'
- 'You mentioned that you really don't like tablets. Tell me, what were you hoping, ideally, that I might be able to do to help?'

Notice the use of softeners such as 'I was just wondering', 'Can I just check with you', 'Tell me' here to make the questions sound more acceptable and less confrontational, and to reduce the likelihood of you getting a tart and unhelpful response.

Define the clinical problem(s)

There are three parts here, each with a single pass criterion.

Obtain additional information about the symptoms and other details of medical history

> 'The doctor obtains sufficient information to include or exclude likely relevant significant conditions.' (P)

The key word here is 'significant', i.e. conditions that might be serious or life threatening, for example:

- a 45-year-old man with musculoskeletal chest pain – you need to have asked enough to exclude an MI
- a 30-year-old woman with breathlessness, just back from a holiday abroad and probably describing a chest infection – you need to have asked enough to exclude a pulmonary embolus
- a small child with a temperature and headache – you need enough information to be able to exclude meningitis.

Assess the patient by appropriate physical and mental examination

> 'The physical/mental examination chosen is likely to confirm or disprove hypotheses that could reasonably have been formed OR is designed to address a patient's concern.' (P)

The examiners will assess the *appropriateness* of what you choose to examine, not the examination itself, which can't really be assessed on video.

Telling the patient what you are going to do (i.e. signposting and getting consent) is helpful to the examiners, as well as being a good consultation skill, for example:

- 'With you having headaches, I'd like to check your blood pressure to see if it's raised.'
- 'Next I'd like to examine your chest to see whether there might be any infection there.'
- 'As you've been dizzy and felt out of breath, I'd like to just check your pulse to see whether your heart is beating regularly.'

Make a working diagnosis

> 'The doctor appears to make a clinically appropriate working diagnosis.' (P)

This is likely to be something that is explained to the patient:

- 'I think you are tired because you might be anaemic. We should check some blood tests and find out.'
- 'Having heard what you've said and listened to your chest, I think you're right; it's likely that you have got a chest infection.'
- 'I know you were worried that this chest pain might be a heart attack but, having listened to what you've told me about the pain and examined you, I'm as sure as I can be that the pain is coming from your ribcage and muscles rather than your heart.'

Explain the problem(s) to the patient

There are two criteria here: sharing the findings with the patient and ensuring that the explanation is understood and accepted by the patient.

Share the findings with the patient

There are both a pass and a merit criterion here.

> 'The doctor explains the problem or diagnosis in appropriate language.' (P)

This means using the patient's vocabulary of nouns, verbs and health language, and avoiding medical language, acronyms and jargon, exactly as you would hope to do in any good consultation.

> 'The doctor's explanation incorporates some or all of the patient's health beliefs.' (M)

This means that, as well as the above, you also incorporate some of the health beliefs that you have already found out by asking what the patient was worried was wrong with them, for example:

- 'I know you were worried about a heart attack, but I'm pleased to be able to say that I really don't think that's the case. Chest pain that is on the left side and made worse by stretching and reaching is really much more likely to be coming from your ribs or muscles.'
- 'You were worried you might have a chest infection, because you had felt feverish and been coughing stuff up and I think you're right – you have.'

Ensure that the explanation is understood and accepted by the patient

> 'The doctor specifically seeks to confirm the patient's understanding of the diagnosis.' (M)

This means more than a cursory 'OK?', 'Got it?' or 'All clear'. What you need to do is find a form of words that works for you and that asks the patient to repeat back to you what you've just said. It seems to work better if this sort of statement incorporates a supposition that if the patient hasn't understood, it is because the doctor has not been sufficiently clear, rather than because the patient is stupid, inattentive or lacking knowledge, etc. Here are some examples:

- 'I know I've told you a lot of information in a short time, so can I just ask you to run through it for me, so that I know you've got it?'
- 'I'm worried I might have confused you with what I said. Can you tell me what you've understood, so that I can clarify any bits that I muddled first time around.'
- 'Now, just repeat back to me, in your own words, what I've said so that we can work out which bits we need to go through in more detail.'

If the patient has mentioned their husband, partner or wife, etc (for example 'I wouldn't have come only the wife was worried and nagged me to do it'), then you have a real gift and a very easy and natural phrase that you can use:

> 'Tell me what you might say when you go home to your husband/wife tonight about what we've been discussing.'

Address the patient's problem(s)

Here there are two criteria, each of them a pass.

Choose an appropriate form of management

> 'The management plan (including any prescription) is appropriate for the working diagnosis, reflecting a good understanding of modern accepted medical practice.' (P)

This is about clinical skills rather than consultation skills and the examiners are looking for whether your management and/or prescribing skills are within the bounds of accepted normal practice.

Involve the patient in the management plan

> 'The patient is given the opportunity to be involved in significant management decisions.' (P)

This is one where a lot of doctors fall down. The criterion means more (much more!) than saying to the patient: 'I'm going to prescribe an antibiotic – is that OK?' or 'Are you OK going for a chest X-ray tomorrow?'

A 'significant' decision is just that. The patient is given enough information to make a real choice about their management, if they wish, for example:

> 'You've had this cough for more than a week and you coughed up some blood this morning. But listening to your chest, there isn't all that much to hear. I think there are several choices here. On the one hand, we could do nothing and see how things go over the next few days and get you to come back if you're not a lot better by the weekend. An antibiotic would be an option, if you wanted to take something for this. I don't think it's likely that the blood you coughed up was anything very significant but, if you are worrying a lot, we could get a quick chest X-ray done. What are your thoughts about this/what would you like to do at the moment?'

Of course, some patients may really not want to be involved in the management decisions, particularly those who grew up in the generation where 'doctor knows best', and it can be quite challenging to help these patients to make informed choices. It is also essential to only give choices that you can live with! If it's clearly a viral infection and you aren't willing to prescribe antibiotics, then don't offer them.

Make effective use of the consultation

And finally, here are two criteria: checking the patient's understanding of the management plan and arranging follow-up of some sort.

> 'The doctor takes steps to enhance concordance by exploring and responding to the patient's understanding of the treatment.' (M)

The 'exploring' part of this is another variant on checking the patient's understanding of the diagnosis and requires the same skills, in other words, finding your own form of words to enable the patient to repeat back to you what you've just said without feeling patronised or belittled. The 'responding' bit is about dealing with what they might say to you! For example:

> **Doctor:** 'I think I may have gone through that rather too quickly. Do you mind if I ask you [softener] to just run through it, so that I'm sure that you've got what I said?'
> **Patient:** 'Err – I'm to take the tablets – one each morning – and see you again in two weeks?' (Doctor notes the slight hesitation both in the 'err' and also in the rising inflexion at the end of the sentence.)
> **Doctor:** 'And the tablets are ...?' (prompting)
> **Patient:** 'Antidepressants.'
> **Doctor:** 'Remember they will take two weeks or so to work. [Reinforcing previous information, and phrasing it positively rather than negatively ('Don't forget to take them for at least two weeks').] How would you explain that to your wife, when you get home?' (Checking understanding by getting the patient to put things into his own words.)

Patient: 'They work on the chemicals in the brain and that can take a while. I've been feeling like this for months. So I can't expect to feel much better overnight.' (Pretty much what the doctor said earlier.)

Doctor: 'Yes, that's a very clear way of putting it. So when you see me in two weeks ...?'

Patient: 'I might not be feeling that much different.'

Doctor: 'That's absolutely right, but you should start to improve soon after that.'

'The doctor specifies the appropriate conditions and interval for follow-up and review.' (P)

This is about safety-netting your consultations with a specific follow-up interval.

- 'I'd expect you to be feeling much better in three or four days but, if you're still coughing then, ring up and come back to see me.'
- 'We should check your blood pressure in about a month. Could you book an appointment with the practice nurse for that?'
- 'I'd like to see you in a fortnight to see how you're feeling but, if you find that your mood seems to be lower, or you or your wife are worried about you, just ring up and come in to see me sooner.'

Videoing consultations – 10 top tips for the MRCGP

- Start videoing as early as you can so that the technical aspects of setting up and using the video become second nature and you are used to the presence of the camera in the room.
- Make sure that your video equipment allows you to see both doctor and patient and that the sound quality is good; this may well mean a wide angle lens and a desk top microphone.
- Learn to structure your consultations well so that you gather all the information you need before you discuss management. It is always difficult if a new piece of significant information emerges very late in the consultation. Summarising every time will help you get this right.
- Practise using rapport and empathy to stand in the patient's shoes and see their problem from their perspective.
- Always ask how the problem is affecting the patient's life – this includes home life, relationships and work.
- Learn to notice cues and practise acknowledging these either straight away or at a suitable moment. If you don't acknowledge cues, the examiners will never know that you noticed them!
- The single most commonly missed criterion is that of offering the patient the opportunity to be involved in significant management decisions. Practise offering choice to patients and make sure that you are willing to let the patient have what they choose.
- When you ask patients about their thoughts and fears, make sure you get an adequate answer. Just asking is not enough! If the answer is superficial, you may need to explore it further.

- If the patient lets something slip out that seems to have dodged the internal policeman, make sure you explore it. A joke or laughter may conceal a real fear that is hard to express.
- In general, one patient with one new problem will give the most straightforward videos. In other words, one patient rather than Mr and Mrs Brown and their children, a single problem rather than a long complex list and a new problem rather than a follow-up. Follow-ups are generally partial consultations with all sorts of assumptions and missing information and it is harder to demonstrate the pass criteria in these.

Possible action points

- Have a look at a video with a colleague and work out where you are now, in terms of the exam.
- If there are particular areas that you consistently tend to miss (common ones are giving the patient the opportunity to be involved in significant management decisions, finding out how the patient's home and work are affected by the problem and specifying the interval for follow-up), you could make a flash card to remind you to practise these in, say, every surgery for a week. If you do this, it will start to become second nature – in other words, incorporated into your unconsciously competent toolkit.

Further reading

- Coles U. *Get Through MRCGP Oral and New Video Modules.* London: Society of Medicine Press Ltd; 2004.
- Tate P. *The Doctor's Communication Handbook.* 5th edn. Oxford: Radcliffe Publishing; 2007.
- www.rcgp.org.uk

Chapter 23

Making a personal learning plan

Key points

- Lifelong learning is the key to both keeping up to date and continued enjoyment of your work in primary care.
- A personal development plan will help you to focus your learning, as well as form part of your annual appraisal.
- It is important to set aims and objectives for your learning.

Introduction

Continuing learning is an essential part of being a primary care practitioner – it is also fun. It needs to be a lifelong process; the day that you stop learning, you might just as well hang up your stethoscope and go home!

A personal learning plan is an effective and efficient way of helping to ensure that you keep up to date and will also be an important part of your appraisal and even revalidation. Planning your learning by using a personal plan, sometimes referred to as personal development plan (PDP), is a very good way of keeping up to date and will help you to take any revalidation process in your stride, rather than it being an insurmountable or overwhelming challenge.

Personal learning plans

Of course, you may well already have a personal learning plan, particularly if you have already taken part in an NHS or other appraisal process. A personal learning plan is a useful and structured way of encapsulating details of learning needs and outcomes. The key stages are:

1. identifying what you need to learn; setting aims and objectives
2. deciding what methods or techniques you will use to achieve this
3. setting a timescale, perhaps with some goals or markers along the way
4. identifying the outcome or change that you will achieve
5. reflecting later on what you have achieved.

Identifying what you need to learn; setting aims and objectives

You may have already decided what you need to learn, perhaps after you have reflected on your work or analysed some consultations. It is important to set aims and objectives. These will help to focus your learning and keep you on track.

Aims

An aim is like the destination of a journey, for example Scarborough.

Objectives

Objectives are the route map that you will use to get there, for example finding out about different routes like rail, bus, road, etc; using a search engine to choose and select a hotel to stay at; telephoning the hotel to book a reservation; checking a map to make sure you know where the hotel is.

In terms of consultation skills, your aim might be, for example, to improve time-keeping in consultations. Your objectives in order to achieve this aim might then be to:

- use the computer system to measure the average length of a consultation both before and after you have implemented your plan
- use summarisation in as many consultations as possible in order to use the time most effectively
- learn to ask patients with lists to prioritise and come back if necessary, in such a way that both you and they feel comfortable with this
- improve your information recording skills, for example by learning to touch-type.

Deciding what methods or techniques you will use to achieve this

If you don't yet know your preferred learning style, find out! Think about your aims and objectives as well as your preferred learning style and work out how best to achieve your objectives, for example:

- reading a book or article on consultation skills
- attending a lecture
- sitting in on a colleague in their surgery and observing
- participating in a seminar on consultation skills, such as 'the naked consultation'
- attending practice-based educational meetings
- working with a group of colleagues to reflect on consultation skills.

For the above example of improving time management in consultations, your methods might include:

- attending a course (touch-typing or time management)
- working with a colleague to look at videos of your consultations and identify areas where you could have used time more efficiently
- practising one small new skill such as summarising in each consultation
- trying out different forms of words to use for patients with lists, so that you can work out which methods are most effective for you.

Timescales

The timescale needs to be realistic. General practice is a long journey and changes to one's behaviour rarely happen overnight. In terms of achieving real change in consultation skills, it is probably reasonable to think in terms of months. This timescale will allow you to revisit what you are doing several times and to work with colleagues to get repeated feedback about your skills. Video analysis will be a particularly useful tool here and you can use it to keep track of your progress and change, and to look back and review your development. With any shorter timescale it may be difficult to achieve lasting change and anything much longer may become endless and never completed.

Identifying the outcome or change

Thinking early on about the changes that you would like to achieve can help to focus your learning and make it specific and realistic. Focusing on the goals is a useful way to shape your learning plan.

Reflecting on changes that you have achieved

Once you have completed a personal learning plan, it may be useful and timely to look back and reflect on what has happened.

- What made you start the plan in the first place?
- Have you achieved what you wanted to achieve?
- Have there been any unexpected pieces of learning?
- Have you been able to work out the methods of learning that work best for you?
- Are there any ways of learning that you now know work less well for you?

Possible action points

- If you have a personal learning plan, get it out now and look at it. Does it still describe what you want to do? Does it need to be updated? If so, do it now!
- If you don't yet have a personal learning plan, use the template in Appendix 2 as a way to start.
- Think what you would like to learn. Be realistic rather than over ambitious. You can always add to the plan as you go along and this is better than being overwhelmed and disheartened.
- Think about your learning style and work out what learning methods will suit you best.

Further reading

- Rughani A. *The GP's Guide to Personal Development Plans*. Oxford: Radcliffe Medical Press; 2000.
- www.londondeanery.ac.uk/gp/downloads/word/nonprincipalpdp.doc
- http://careerfocus.bmjjournals.com/cgi/content/full/325/7358/S36

Conclusion

General practice today is in a state of flux as never before. Perhaps the only real certainty about the future is that there will continue to be change. But whatever organisational changes lie ahead, it is very likely that the consultation between health professional and patient will remain the cornerstone of primary care. Good consultation skills undoubtedly help patients to feel better during the process of consultation but they are just as rewarding for the health professional as the patient. Every consultation provides opportunities for learning and practising skills, because each patient that we see is different from every other patient. Continued learning and development of consultation skills are just as important as keeping up to date with guidelines, new drugs, 'best practice', etc and will help you to enrich your consultations as well as help you to continue to enjoy general practice and avoid burnout or disillusionment.

Having read this far, I hope that you now have the tools and techniques that you need to help with your consultation skills and it is my sincere wish that, above all, you will now enjoy more of your consultations, more of the time!

Jargon buster

Anchoring	A useful NLP technique that enables people to associate touching part of their body (e.g. hand or face) with particular feelings (e.g. confidence, happiness). The feeling is said to be anchored to the body part. It is easy to learn and easy to teach to patients.
Auditory predicate	Listen for hearing words such as 'He said to me ... and then I said to him ...'. A patient who uses these sorts of words primarily experiences the world through what they hear, rather than through what they see or touch. By matching your language to theirs, you can help them more effectively.
Authentic feelings	In transactional analysis, four authentic feelings are described: sad, mad (angry), glad (happy) and scared. Any other feelings such as guilt, embarrassment, jealousy, helplessness are 'racket' feelings and are concealing one of the authentic feelings.
Balint groups	There are a number of these groups around the country. A group of six to eight doctors commit to meeting weekly for a long period (at least one to two years) with a psychotherapist to facilitate. Members of the group bring problems that they have encountered with managing patients, particularly those with psychological problems. The group and the facilitator help members to gain insight into the issues. It should be noted that these are not 'therapy groups' for doctors.
Body language	Communicating via the musculoskeletal system rather than with words; often more significant than verbal language. The way that we sit, stand, move or look communicates volumes about how we are feeling inside. The intuitive clinician pays attention to their own body language as well as being very aware of what patients are communicating with theirs.
Catharsis	An emotional release – often tears or uncontrollable laughter or trembling; usually very helpful in helping to move patients forward.
CBT	Cognitive Behavioural Therapy. A technique of brief therapy often used by psychologists.

	It is based on the principle that if thinking and feeling are linked, then changing the (conscious) thinking can change the (unconscious) feelings. This type of therapy is very useful for patients with difficulties that are fairly clear and specific, e.g. panic attacks, agoraphobia. It aims to help patients solve problems rather than change their personality.
Calibration	Working out what representational systems are used by someone else. You can do this by paying attention to the language that patients are using as well as watching their tiny eye movements as they are talking to you or responding to your questions. For example, if you ask them to remember something they have heard (a conversation or something that was said to them by someone else), you might observe their eyes flicking left or right (usually left) and in a horizontal plane compared with their eyes (i.e. neither up nor down).
Chunk and check	Useful when giving information to patients. Give it in manageable chunks and check understanding before giving any more.
Closed questions	Questions which can be answered with 'yes' or 'no', e.g. 'Have you lost weight?' These questions can be useful for clarifying specific details but are less effective than open questions during the early part of a consultation because they tend to stop the patient telling their story.
Cognitive dissonance	An unsettling state of inner conflict or distress when what we are experiencing of the world out there no longer fits our internal model of it. It is a powerful tool for change.
Connect	The first stage of the Neighbour model. Engaging with patients and developing rapport with them.
Counter-transference	The feelings that arise in a health professional during a consultation that are actually coming from the patient. Awareness of these and the ability to feed them back to the patient can be a very effective way of moving difficult consultations forward. For example, the 'heartsink' patient seems to have an endless list of insoluble problems. The doctor or nurse starts to feel frustrated and overwhelmed. Instead of becoming irritated, they recognise that these feelings (which they didn't have before the patient walked in) are actually coming from the

	patient and gently offer an interpretation to the patient, 'I'm wondering if you're feeling frustrated and a bit overwhelmed with all this'.
Curtain raisers	A very spontaneous opening of a consultation by a patient, e.g. 'Gosh this is a big room – I usually see Dr Smith, you know.'
Deletions	One of the three types of speech censoring. The patient says something but essential details are missing, e.g. 'No one understands', 'It's no better', 'I'm really worried about her', 'It started a year ago'.
Displacement	Of feelings. The patient who is angry with you may actually be angry with someone else or frustrated with themselves. The feelings are displaced onto you. Recognising this can help you to get to the bottom of the patient's real problem rather than getting upset or responding defensively to the patient.
Distortions	One of the types of speech censoring (along with deletions and generalisations). The patient turns a behaviour or action into a noun or even an abstract concept, e.g. 'I don't like his attitude', 'I'm suffering from stress', 'I need help'.
Doctor as drug	Another of Michael Balint's phrases. The interaction between doctor and patient is therapeutic in its own right. Many patients do not need a prescription for drugs but most of them need time and attention and will get better faster because you give them this.
Doctor-centred	Who does most of the talking in your consultations? Doctor-centred consultations may miss the patient's real worries or agenda.
'Don't' means 'do'	The right half of the brain doesn't hear the words 'not' or 'don't'. So if you say 'it won't hurt', the patient hears that it might. If you say 'Don't forget to complete the course of tablets', the right side of the brain hears that you could forget, etc. Express it positively, e.g. 'You'll just feel me touching', 'Finish all the tablets'.
Ego state	Described by Eric Berne. At any moment each of us is in the parent, adult or child mode. This is most apparent in the way that we interact with other people.

- Parent – nurturing, caring, controlling, making judgements
- Adult – analysing, processing information, interacting with the outside world
- Child – free, creative, spontaneous, trying to please

	The most effective consultations with patients are adult–adult transactions, not parent–child.
Empathy	Being in tune with the patient; stepping into their shoes and feeling how it is for them.
Eye contact	Looking at the patient when they're speaking to you and when you're speaking to them (rather than looking away at the computer). This is very important for helping to build and maintain rapport.
Eye movements	Watch the patient's tiny eye movements when they are talking to you. If their eyes move upwards, they're remembering or constructing something visual; horizontal movements indicate auditory memories; and downward ones demonstrate kinaesthetic experiences or internal search. This can help you work out whether a patient's preferred representational system is visual, auditory or kinaesthetic.
Gambits	A set-piece opener that has been prepared by a patient before a consultation, e.g. 'I hope I'm not wasting your time doctor but ....'
Games People Play	Excellent book by Eric Berne. Describes the games that patients and clinicians unconsciously play in consultations, including: NIGYSOB (Now I've got you, son of a bitch); ITHY (I'm only trying to help you); SWYMMD (See what you made me do); YDYB ('Why don't you ...?', 'Yes, but ...'); 'Ain't it awful ...'. It's well worth (re)reading and noting how many of the different games are played out in your consulting room. Recognising the games can enable you to stop being an unconscious participant and to help the patient to move forward.
Generalisations	One of the three types of speech censoring, it tends to include the words 'always', 'never', 'every', e.g. 'No one understands me', 'I can't take tablets', 'I hate hospitals', 'All psychiatrists are rubbish'.
Gestalt counselling	'Gestalt' is a German word meaning 'whole', in the sense of more than the sum of the parts. Gestalt counselling pays attention to feelings, thoughts, sensations and fantasies, helping people to recognise behaviour that may be limiting a sense of wholeness or satisfaction and enabling them to change.
Gift wrapping	A term coined by Roger Neighbour to describe the way that a management plan can most effectively be presented to a patient, in a way that is both transparent and attractive.

Hand-over	The fourth of the five stages of Roger Neighbour's model of the consultation. This stage is about sharing the management plan with the patient.
Hesitations	A type of speech censoring and a sign of cognitive dissonance. The patient who has been speaking quite fluently starts to hesitate and to include 'um', 'er', 'well', 'I mean', 'sort of'.
Housekeeping	The fifth and final stage of the Neighbour model. This is an internal check for the doctor that they are in good shape to deal with the next consultation. It also refers to steps that doctors take long term to look after themselves.
Inner Consultation, The	Roger Neighbour's classic book on the consultation.
Inner Apprentice, The	Neighbour's follow-up to *The Inner Consultation*, describing skills and techniques to improve the trainer–GP registrar relationship and teaching.
Internal search	The patient breaks eye contact and is looking down and concentrating. They are internally processing something and it can be helpful not to interrupt their thought flow by talking. When they resurface, it is likely to be with something significant – don't miss it.
Kinaesthetic predicate	A preference for processing the world through touching and feeling. Watch and listen for touching and feeling words – both physical and emotional, e.g. 'You could have knocked me down with a feather'.
Locus	Latin for 'place'. In consultation terminology, this is used to express the place where the power or control is in the consultation at any given moment, e.g. with the doctor or the patient, or at any place between them, nearer to one than the other.
Magical thinking	Remember when you were six and didn't dare step on the cracks in the pavement in case the bears jumped out at you? This is magical thinking. Patients faced with a serious diagnosis can enter the realm of magical thinking, e.g. 'If only I lose weight/stop smoking/follow the doctor's instructions to the letter, then everything will be alright/my cancer will be cured.'
Maslow's pyramid	Of hierarchical needs. Abraham Maslow described a hierarchy of human needs starting with basic safety needs at the bottom (food, warmth, shelter) and moving up through friendship and trust to self-fulfilment at the top

	of the pyramid. At any moment, each individual is most concerned with their lowest unfilled needs and can move down or up the pyramid at any time. If an individual becomes ill, their needs move right down the pyramid to a very low level.
Michael Balint	Author of the classic book, *The Doctor, His Patient and the Illness*. This was the first work to recognise and state that doctors have feelings in consultations and that acknowledgement and recognition of them can help the doctor to perform more effectively.
Milton Erickson	An American master-therapist who first described the 'My friend John' technique. Confined to a wheelchair by polio, he was a charismatic teacher and enormously effective psychotherapist.
Minimal cues	Information about what's going on inside the patient leaks out. Minimal cues are tiny behaviours that doctors and nurses recognise in patients (and, similarly, patients recognise in their doctors or nurses) that give insight into the inner workings of each others' minds.
Minimal encouragers	The way that we encourage patients to continue to tell their story with, e.g. 'yes', 'mm, mm', 'I see', 'go on'. This includes non-verbal ways such as nodding and looking attentive as well.
Mutual investment company	A term coined by Michael Balint to describe the fact that general practice consultations can extend over a period of years and that clinician and patient both invest time and trust into the relationship.
'My friend John'	A useful way of engaging the attention of patients and offering suggestions or interpretations in a non-threatening way. 'Something like this happened to my friend John (or another patient or someone I know, etc) and he was just as worried as you are, but in fact ... happened, and all was well', etc. 'My friend John' puts a slight distance between the patient and their possible anxieties, so that they can easily choose either to identify with 'John' or to say that it doesn't apply to them. First described by Milton Erickson.
NLP	Neurolinguistic programming. A set of skills and techniques that enable helpers to work very effectively with their clients.
Non-sequiturs	When something a patient says just doesn't follow on from what they've just said (knight's

move thinking). It indicates that great chunks may have been left out and is a sign of cognitive dissonance. It is worth exploring further.

Non-verbal skills

The way that you stand, sit, move, etc speaks volumes about you. In other words, this is how you communicate with your musculoskeletal system rather than your voice. Skilled clinicians ensure that their non-verbal skills are honed as skilfully as their verbal skills.

Omissions

A type of speech censoring. Very important and specific details are left out so that the listener has to ask for more information in order to make sense of what the patient's just said. It's worth exploring but also worth noting exactly how you feel when the patient does this. (*See* counter-transference.)

Open questions

Ones where the patient can't answer 'yes' or 'no', e.g. 'Tell me how you've been sleeping lately'. These questions tend to yield much more information than closed questions.

Patient-centred

The other end of the spectrum from doctor-centred. The locus, or 'place', of the consultation is with the patient. The doctor is chiefly concerned with helping the patient to express their symptoms, fears, expectations, etc rather than following their own doctor-centred agenda.

Patient's health beliefs

All patients have ideas, concerns and expectations when they come to see you. You need to find out what they are. One model (Helman) suggests that all patients have six questions:
- What has happened?
- Why has it happened?
- Why has it happened to me?
- Why now?
- What would happen if I do nothing about it?
- What should I do or whom should I see for further advice?

Pendleton model

A seven-stage model of the consultation developed by David Pendleton.

Peak experiences

Described by Abraham Maslow. Moments when an individual experiences profound love, joy, fulfilment, understanding or happiness. Self-actualising people experience more of these moments than others and also tend to focus on problems outside themselves, being creative, spontaneous and not too bound by social convention.

Pendleton's rules	A safe way of giving feedback when looking at consultation videos. Briefly: the person being watched goes first; good points first; recommendations for change rather than criticisms.
Predicates	A person's preferred way of processing information about the world around them. This can be visual, auditory or kinaesthetic.
Presuppositions	A shepherding technique. If you really want a patient to do A, then you ask them to do B, where B can only be done if you've done A first, e.g. if I want you to read this lexicon, then rather than say 'Read it' I might ask you to tell me what you think of the contents, making the presupposition that you will have read it first. In consultations: 'Telephone me in a week's time after you've completed the course of tablets to let me know how you're feeling' presupposes: 'You will take the tablets for a week' or 'Would you find it easier to stop smoking all at once or to cut down gradually over a month?' presupposes 'You will stop smoking!'
Racket feelings	A term used in transactional analysis. These are feelings that are displayed by people who have learnt them in childhood. Some people, for example, translate most of their emotions into anger. So they appear to be cross or angry when their real feeling is sadness or fear.
Rapport	An active process that has to be constantly worked on throughout the consultation. It describes the state in which two people are mutually responsive to each others' signals.
Representational system	Visual, auditory or kinaesthetic. The preferred mode in which any individual tends to process information about the world around them.
Reframing	You can't always alter the situation, but you can sometimes help a patient to feel differently, and better, about it by nudging their imagination. Remember how Tom Sawyer persuaded his friends to whitewash the fence for him (*see* p. 88).
Reflection	Repeating back to a patient what they have just said to you. Although this may feel artificial at first, you will find that patients do not perceive it like that and that they feel listened to and understood.
Rogerian counselling	Person-centred counselling, developed by Carl Rogers.

Roger Neighbour	A GP and former Course Organiser from Abbots Langley who developed an intuitive five-stage model of the consultation: connect, summarise, handover, safety net, housekeeping.
Rubber bands	In TA terms, the elastic that pulls people back to their racket feelings.
Safety-netting	The fourth stage of the Neighbour model. Explaining to the patient what you expect to happen, how you'll know if you're right or wrong and what action the patient should then take.
Semi-closed questions	Ones that can't be answered with 'yes' or 'no' but nevertheless can be answered with a fairly brief and not very illuminating answer, e.g. 'How many times do you need to get up in the night?'; answer – 1, 2, 3 etc.
Shepherding	Using value-laden phrases to influence patients, e.g. you could give a patient information about HRT by saying, 'The latest evidence suggests that it's much more harmful than we first thought' or 'There is a small risk of developing breast cancer if you take HRT but a definite risk of osteoporosis causing fractures if you don't take it.'
Signposting	Telling the patient what you are going to do, rather than just going ahead and doing it. In other words, you are thinking aloud and sharing this with them, e.g. 'In a moment I'd like to examine you, but before I do that I'd like to ...', 'I just need to look at the computer for a few moments to check what investigations you've had'. This helps patients to feel more in control of the consultation as equal partners in it, and less like vulnerable children.
Somatisation	Some patients are somatisers. They experience their emotions as physical symptoms. The doctor or nurse who keeps investigating and treating these symptoms will find that the patients continue to return, because their (unconscious) emotional needs have not been satisfactorily addressed. This behaviour has often been learnt in childhood – only physical symptoms get parental interest and attention.
Speech censoring	When something is clearly being left out. There might be hesitations, prevarications, generalisations, omissions, distortions or non-sequiturs. A coded signal that indicates cognitive dissonance. All is not as it appears and it is often worth probing a bit deeper.

Summarise	One of the most useful techniques in the consultation. When in doubt about where to go or what to do next – summarise! The second stage of the Neighbour consultation model. By this stage you have enough information to summarise clearly back to the patient the reasons why they have come to see you, their own thoughts and their expectations of the consultation.
TA	Transactional analysis. A type of therapy first described by Eric Berne, it is a way of looking at what goes on inside people and in relationships between people. (*See* Ego state.)
Transference	A term used to describe the development of strong feelings by a patient towards their doctor, nurse, therapist, etc.
Value-laden phrases	Values are the choices that we make under pressure. Listen for the patient's values when they're talking to you and remember that the words that we use to describe behaviours or actions can make it more or less likely that the patient will do what we want.
Visual predicate	This is the commonest type of predicate. Most people primarily experience the world around them through what they see, rather than what they hear or touch. Listen for the patient using descriptive or visual words like 'I see what you mean' and match your language to theirs for maximum effectiveness.
Who is the patient?	A phrase coined by Michael Balint. When there is more than one 'patient' in a consultation, it can be helpful to try and work out which one is actually the real one. It's not always the one you think, e.g. a young mum presents her baby as being ill, unsettled or not sleeping, but actually it's the mum who's depressed or not coping well and needs help. Treating the baby or just reassuring the mum will not deal with the whole problem.
Yes set	This means that the patient is in agreement with everything you have just said, e.g. when you have summarised back to the patient and got it all right and they have nothing more they think they need to tell you. If they say 'Yes, but ...' in any shape or form, you haven't yet reached a 'yes set'. Remember, if you haven't got a yes, you've got a 'no'.

Some useful resources

Sample consent form for videoing consultations

(easily adaptable for audio recording)

PATIENT CONSENT TO VIDEO RECORDING FOR ASSESSMENT PURPOSES

Date ....

Patient's name ....

Name(s) of person(s) accompanying patient ....

....

- Dr/Nurse ...., who you are seeing today, is hoping to make video recordings of some consultations.
- The video is ONLY of you and the doctor or nurse talking together. Intimate examinations will not be recorded and the camera will be switched off at any time if you wish. All video recordings are carried out according to guidelines issued by the General Medical Council.
- The video will only be used for learning and teaching purposes and possibly for research and quality control. The tape will be securely stored and is subject to the same degree of confidentiality as your medical records. The tape will be erased as soon as practicable and in any event within three years.
- The security and confidentiality of the video recording are the responsibility of the doctor or nurse.
- You do not have to agree to your consultation with the doctor being recorded. If you do not want your consultation to be recorded, please tell Reception. This is not a problem and will not affect your consultation in any way. But if you do not mind your consultation being recorded, we are grateful to you. If you wish, you may view the tape recording before confirming your consent.
- If you consent to this consultation being recorded, please sign where shown below.

Thank you very much for your help.

TO BE COMPLETED BY THE PATIENT

I have read and understood the above information and give my permission for my consultation to be video recorded.

.... Date ....

Signature of the patient BEFORE THE CONSULTATION

.... Date ....
Signature(s) of any person(s) accompanying the patient

After seeing the doctor I am still willing/I no longer wish my consultation to be used for the above purposes.

.... Date ....
Signature of patient AFTER THE CONSULTATION

.... Date ....
Signature(s) of any person(s) accompanying the patient

Consultation log

This log is a tool to help you to record and identify consultations that cause you stress or difficulty.

Which patient?	Were you in good shape?	What happened?	How did you feel?	Any other observations or comments

Personal development template

What development needs do I have? (Explain the need)	How will I address them? (Explain how you will take action and what resources you will need)	Date by which I plan to achieve development goal (Date)	Outcome (How will your practice change as a result of the development activity?)	Completed (Date and time taken)

Index

Page numbers in *italic* refer to figures or tables.